NORTH CAROLINA &
THE PROBLEM OF AIDS

NORTH CAROLINA &
THE PROBLEM OF AIDS

Advocacy, Politics, & Race in the South

STEPHEN INRIG

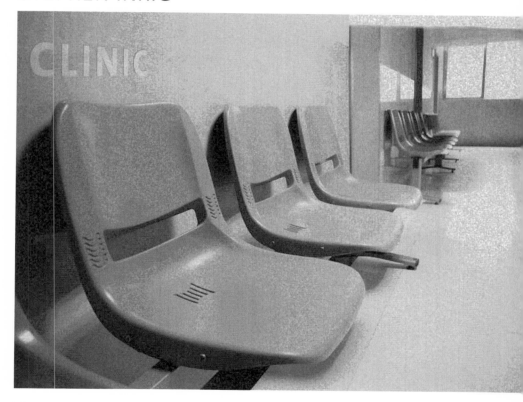

The University of North Carolina Press   Chapel Hill

Manufactured in the United States of America

Set in Whitman and Univers

The paper in this book meets the guidelines for permanence and durability of the Committee on Production Guidelines for Book Longevity of the Council on Library Resources.

The University of North Carolina Press has been a member of the Green Press Initiative since 2003.

Library of Congress Cataloging-in-Publication Data
Inrig, Stephen.
   North Carolina and the problem of AIDS : advocacy,
   politics, and race in the South / Stephen Inrig.
      p. cm.
   Includes bibliographical references and index.
   ISBN 978-0-8078-3498-5 (hardback : alk. paper)
   ISBN 978-1-4696-1883-8 (pbk. : alk. paper)
   1. AIDS (Disease)—North Carolina—History.
   2. AIDS (Disease)—Social aspects—North Carolina. 3. AIDS
   (Disease)—Southern States—History. 4. African American
   gays—Diseases. I. Title.
   RA643.84.N8157 2011
   362.196'9792009756—dc23
                          2011025920

cloth   15 14 13 12 11   5 4 3 2 1
paper 18 17 16 15 14   5 4 3 2 1

THIS BOOK WAS DIGITALLY PRINTED.

For Jula

CONTENTS

FIGURES AND TABLES

Figures

Tables

ACKNOWLEDGMENTS

I have many people to thank for making this book possible. I owe intellectual and professional debts to several people. Margaret Humphreys, my key adviser during my time at Duke, patiently directed an often unconventional student as I navigated my graduate experience at Duke, and her support has continued to open doors of opportunity to me that would not be opened otherwise. She read some of the earliest iterations of the manuscript, and I appreciated her humor, candor, and ever-present generosity throughout this process. Along with Margaret, Peter English provided hours of support during my time at Duke, and I left there with not only the skills he taught but also the indelible marks of graciousness and friendship that he left on my life. Finally, the work and friendship of James Thomas, at the University of North Carolina–Chapel Hill, has proved profoundly influential on the way I view disease, society, and the endeavor for social justice in this world. Jim has also modeled what it means to be an intellectually engaged person of faith, for which I am truly thankful.

I started this project when I was at Duke, refined it at UNC, and completed it at my present home at the University of Texas Southwestern Medical Center in Dallas. I have many people at each institution to thank for their help along the way. At Duke, John Thompson and Robin Ennis enabled me to finish my graduate studies ahead of schedule. Other academic mentors, including Jeffrey Baker, Susan Thorne, Claudia Koonz, and William Chafe, were generous with their time and insights. UNC's Center for the Study of the American South supported me as a postdoctoral fellow in Southern Studies during 2007 and 2008. I thank Dr. Harry Watson and the staff there for providing me with a wonderful fellowship that allowed me the time and support I needed to conduct the major oral history portion of this project and to begin writing this book. My department chair at UT, Dr. Milton Packer, has been enormously supportive, and my division chief, Dr. John Sadler, has provided tremendous support, guidance, and encouragement in my recent endeavors. I am grateful for the support of all my divisional colleagues and staff, and I am particularly indebted to Dr. Simon Craddock Lee for numerous keen insights as I worked to shape the last parts of this book.

The origins of this book stem from my time working with Duke's Promising Practices Youth Program. That program would not have existed save for the strong advocacy of Duke University Health System's then-chancellor, Dr. Ralph Snyderman; vice chancellor, Dr. Jean Spaulding; and associate vice president, MaryAnn Black. I owe each of them a debt of gratitude for providing me with flexible leave to pursue my doctorate degree and to share the findings in my study with my students. I am also deeply grateful to the students and families who allowed me into their lives during my time running the Promising Practices Youth Program. I have written this book to answer those hard questions they kept asking. I hope this book helps them find some answers. And, by the way, a black man *can* become president.

Most of the archival research for this project was done at the Duke University Rare Book, Manuscript, and Special Collections Library, and the staff there provided me hours of exceptional assistance as I did work in the archives of various AIDS Service Organizations. I would particularly like to thank Jodi Berkowitz, Melissa Delbridge, Elizabeth Dunn, Megan Lewis, Linda McCurdy, Laura Micham, Nixie Miller, Eleanor Mills, Janie Morris, Ali Poffinberger, and Kelly Wooten. I owe to Ian Lekus, who now teaches history at Harvard, an extra note of gratitude, as he originally catalogued and organized many of the files that provided me with research material. He was also very generous in providing the transcripts of many of his oral histories of Lesbian and Gay Health Project members. The oral history project at UNC's Center for the Study of the American South was also of great help, and I appreciate the work that Jacquelyn Dowd Hall, David Cline, and others have done with that program over the years. I also want to thank the staff of the North Carolina Department of Statistics for providing me information on incarceration rates, county AIDS reports, and the like. The oral history respondents themselves were profoundly generous with their time, particularly David Jolly, Dante Noto, Anthony Adinolfi, Louise Alston, Howard Fitts, and Richard Rumley, and I am grateful to them.

A number of graduate colleagues supported me through this process, either through their friendship or through the reading of my wretched material (and I trust through both). I am particularly grateful to Timothy Schulz and Benjamin Grob-Fitzgibbon for their friendship and fellowship, and I am forever indebted to my writing group—Kelly Kennington, Sebastian Lukasik, Gordon Mantler, and Michael Weisel—for their friendship and their relentless patience reading the early drafts of the book. I should also thank friends who proved needed distractions from my work during this time, including

Nat Stine, Rachel Stine, Tom Fletcher, Eric Laycock, Tim O'Brien, Dan Yarbrough, John Booth, Heather Isfan, and Daniel and Krista Marcy.

The University of North Carolina Press has proved a valuable partner in guiding me through the publication process. Mary Caviness provided excellent editorial wisdom and guidance in the final stages of this book, and I am deeply grateful for all her outstanding suggestions and superb advice. David Perry and Sian Hunter also provided excellent observations, suggestions, insights, and exhortations. This book is certainly better owing to their help.

Finally, I must acknowledge the profound support of my family in this process. Two of my three children were born during this effort, and for much of the time, I served as a stay-at-home father while I worked on it. Evan, McKenna, and Lawson, I love you with all my heart, and consider my time with you as my number one responsibility; this is my "other" job. My parents and in-laws have provided tremendous help in this process, as well, reading and editing my various chapters and flying across country to watch the kids for a week so I could go sit in a coffee shop and write. Deb, thank you for all your help with the writing and with watching the kids. Chuck, thanks for the humor and the constant donation of your wife and your time so I could finish the book. Mom, thank you for child care support and heartfelt encouragement all along the way. Dad, thank you for reading every word of this document and saving me from some embarrassing mistakes. All of you have modeled academic excellence, personal integrity, and sacrificial discipleship my whole life; I am grateful for your investment in my life. Lastly, I owe my deepest gratitude to my wife, Jula, who has encouraged and prodded me throughout this process. Jula, you have supported me through this all and put up with all the late-night studying and messy stacks of books. I know that your love for me is the deepest and best part of my life, and I thank you for all the ways you made this happen. I dedicate this book to you.

NORTH CAROLINA &
THE PROBLEM OF AIDS

IN A PLACE SO ORDINARY

The Problem of AIDS in North Carolina and the American South

In February 2003, North Carolina's Screening and Tracing of Active Transmission (STAT) team learned of two black college men who tested positive for "acute" HIV infections. After an initial HIV infection, it can take several weeks for the body to make antibodies. During this "acute" phase of infection, individuals are at their most contagious owing to a high viral load, but since standard HIV tests only detect antibodies to the virus, they often fail to detect infections in the acute phase. In the mid-1990s, researchers developed tests called nucleic acid amplification tests (NAAT) that could target nucleic acid sequences specific to HIV, allowing them to identify HIV infection at much earlier stages. By November 2002, North Carolina had established a team that performed NAAT tests on all new HIV-infected blood samples from publicly funded venues.[1] It was this team that uncovered the acute infections in the two college men.

These results caught the STAT team off guard: while they knew college students acquired HIV, they had not considered "colleges as hot spots for transmissions." Indeed, the team realized they knew very little about how frequently seroconversions occurred among college students in North Carolina, and they set out to explain what was going on. Were these just incidental findings, common occurrences, or signs of a new trend? What the team uncovered was a mini-outbreak of HIV among college students in and around Raleigh and Durham. The particulars of the outbreak were unique: of the twenty-eight college men who had acquired HIV in the Raleigh-Durham area in the previous three years, most were black, most had sex with men, and most attended historically black colleges. In August 2004, the Centers for Disease Control and Prevention (CDC) published the results of the STAT team's investigation in its *Morbidity and Mortality Weekly Report (MMWR)*.[2]

At the time this report was published, I was a graduate student in the history of medicine at Duke University with a particular interest in the history of AIDS. I has also just taken paternity leave from my job as director of a mentoring project for at-risk children and adolescents in Durham, North Carolina. Part of my work with the project involved pairing disadvantaged but academically gifted high school students with doctors and medical students at Duke University School of Medicine. I also spent time with the students teaching them various life skills and healthy behaviors. Several of my students were African Americans, many planned on attending historically black colleges in the state, and at least two of them were gay. So when, in the course of my graduate research, this article caught my eye, I immediately thought of "my kids." The truth was my students had seen a lot of life. Many of my students were sexually active, some had contact with gangs, and at least one was pregnant. We talked very openly about their private lives.

I wondered what they would make of this study when I spent time with them later. Since I was writing letters for their college applications, I knew my gay students would ask me directly whether they should reconsider going to historically black colleges. The rest would ask more general questions, like why black men in North Carolina's black colleges were at greater risk for HIV than others. These questions were only compounded in the ensuing months, after the CDC released a second report on high rates of HIV among local women, "HIV Transmission among Black Women—North Carolina, 2004."[3] These studies prompted the expected questions and several others when I broached them with my students and with others. How large a problem was HIV/AIDS among African Americans in North Carolina, everyone wanted to know. Moreover, if the problem was as dire as these CDC reports suggested, how had HIV/AIDS become such a problem? When I had discussed AIDS with my students, I largely referenced San Francisco, New York City, crack houses, or Africa; we never considered that a rampant AIDS epidemic might exist among African Americans in North Carolina. And yet here we were, with some of my students worried about what they might find when they started college the following year. How had things gotten this way, they wanted to know, and what was being done about it? At the time, I did not have any good answers. This study is an attempt to answer their questions.

To begin with, I had to explore what it was about the North Carolina AIDS reports that surprised me. I was not unaware of the problem of AIDS: I had made my first donation to a domestic AIDS organization back in the late 1980s, I routinely taught "safe sex" to the kids in my program, and I was also concerned about AIDS in Africa. Yet I had assumed the American AIDS epidemic still to be a problem of white gay men in major urban centers, especially on the coasts. The North Carolina data could be an outlier, I reasoned, or I might have to recalibrate my understanding of AIDS in America.

Four interrelated paradigms influenced the way I viewed the AIDS epidemic in this country, and these were the major themes I had used when I taught the history of AIDS to my undergraduate students. The first major theme guiding my perspective is what I call the "tragic gay heroism" model. Randy Shilts's chronicle of the epidemic's early years, *And the Band Played On*, formed the baseline source material for this theme, though I supplemented it with other works like Andrew Holleran's novel *Ground Zero*, Larry Kramer's *Reports from the Holocaust*; media and theatrical representations like Larry Kramer's *The Normal Heart*, Norman Rene's *Longtime Companion*, Peter Friedman and Tom Joslin's *Silverlake Life*, and Tony Kushner's *Angels in America*; and Paul Monette's moving AIDS memoir, *Borrowed Time*.[4] This paradigm focuses on the tragic heroism of gay men in San Francisco, New York, and Washington in their effort to overcome denial and discrimination and to confront the Reagan administration to force action against AIDS while protecting themselves from the devastation it wrought. My baseline assumption about AIDS in the United States was that it had largely started with and disproportionately affected white gay men in places like New York and San Francisco, and that much of what the United States had done to attack the problem of AIDS — whether that meant investment in medical research or in "safer sex" initiatives — were the result of gay men's efforts.

Closely related to this paradigm was a second one, what I call "the battle for AIDS exceptionalism." This model portrayed AIDS policy battles as a struggle between the forces of rationality and compassion and the forces of fear and moralistic discrimination. The work of Shilts and Kramer clearly fit into this model, as did the stories about school-aged children and their families, like Ryan White and his mother, who were hounded out of their schools and communities by intolerant school boards, irrational parents, and petrified children.[5] The guiding work for me in this paradigm was Ronald Bayer's *Private Acts, Social Consequences*, which investigated the early policy battles waged between public health professionals and gay communities over the balance between individual rights and public health in San Francisco and New York.[6] In this and later works, Bayer drew attention to the unique cluster of approaches, known as AIDS exceptionalism, that AIDS activists and their allies used to address the epidemic. According to Bayer, AIDS exceptionalism was "a commitment to rely on prevention measures that were noncoercive — that respect the privacy and social rights of those who were at risk. Mass education, voluntary testing, and counseling were at the center of a public health strategy that sought to avoid interventions that might 'drive the epidemic underground.'"[7] Central to this exceptionalist paradigm was the idea of patient-initiated or client-initiated testing, that is, that testing should be a voluntary decision largely initiated by the patient or client, rather than by the medical professional. Along with patient-initiated testing, AIDS exceptionalism included explicit consent of those tested, strong confidentiality protections, if not anonymity, and robust pre- and post-test counseling. The testing and counseling protections associated with AIDS exceptionalism were frequently bundled together under the rubric of Voluntary Counseling and Testing (VCT).[8]

A third paradigm informing my perspective on AIDS in America was what I call "the changing face of AIDS" model. In the late 1980s and early 1990s, AIDS rates in white gay communities stabilized and began declining, while AIDS rates continued climbing among women, minorities, children, and adolescents. "The face of AIDS in America is changing," *Time* magazine proclaimed in 1987; "it is getting younger, darker, more feminine."[9] "As the disease spreads more rapidly among heroin users and their sexual partners," Ronald Bayer argued in 1989, "the color of those who fall victim will darken even further."[10] Dysfunction among minorities and women played an important role in this paradigm: many stories focused on the intractable problem of black drug users acquiring the virus while sharing needles in crack houses, while women were "relegated to the drug abuser category, or partners of drug abusers, or the supremely negative category of bad mother . . . 'unruly,' 'chaotic,' and 'despairing.'"[11] Also prominent in this model were the disclosures from prominent African Americans—like Max Robinson, Magic Johnson, and Arthur Ashe—of their HIV/AIDS status. Frequently these disclosures devolved into debates about black male sexuality, and they fed into a secondary discourse around black men on the "down low," which hit the "Oprah" circuit in the late 1990s and early 2000s and served as a key explanation for the disproportionate impact of AIDS on black communities.[12]

The final paradigm that informed my viewpoint on AIDS was the "march of medical progress" model. The underlying assumption in this model was that biomedicine could solve the technical problems associated with HIV and would eventually find a cure (or at least a long-term therapy). The journey toward this assumption was not without its drama, of course, and so considerable attention was paid to the biases of early researchers, the search for the virus, and the long struggle to find an acceptable therapy or effective vaccine.[13] Important in this discussion was the ambivalent, often confrontational, relationship between AIDS activists and AIDS clinical researchers, including the herculean effort made by feminists to include more women and minorities in clinical research.[14] The underlying message in each of these stories was that a great deal of progress had already been made in prevention (condoms and needle exchange) and therapy (Highly Active Antiretroviral Therapy [HAART]), and that scientists would continue to find effective prevention models, prophylactics, and therapies, and, one day, a cure, ideally avoiding politics, bureaucracy, moralism, and ideology in the process.

While the epidemic in North Carolina did not strictly contradict these paradigms, it did complicate them. Unsurprisingly, AIDS in North Carolina disproportionately affected African Americans: in 2004, the rate of HIV infection for African Americans was eight times higher than for Caucasians; the rate for black men was almost seven times higher than for white men; and the rate for black women was fourteen times higher than for white women.[15] What was surprising was that HIV had disproportionately affected African Americans in the state from the very beginning of the epidemic; in 1985, African Americans already accounted for more cases of AIDS than Caucasians, even though they constituted only about a quarter of the population. The face of AIDS had indeed changed in North Carolina, but it had not really followed the "white to black" pattern suggested by the narrative in other communities. Furthermore, HIV in North Carolina was surprisingly rural: since at least the early 1990s, about 25 percent of North Carolina's HIV disease reports had consistently come from rural counties; indeed, some of those counties reported the highest HIV infection rates in the state, and, nationally, North Carolina itself had the second highest number of AIDS cases coming from rural areas.[16] North Carolina's experience of rural AIDS complicated the urban/inner-city model gleaned from other parts of the country. Finally, reports about new HIV/AIDS cases had remained relatively stable in the state since the mid-1990s, while the proportion of people infected increasingly skewed toward African Americans and other minorities. Whatever therapies and evidence-based interventions were improving AIDS acquisition and care in Caucasian communities were having less impact in North Carolina.

Moreover, these epidemiological "peculiarities" were not confined to North Carolina: other southern states reported similar data with respect to HIV/AIDS.[17] Consequently, by 2007, the South reported the greatest proportion of new AIDS diagnoses in the nation (46 percent), the greatest proportion of people estimated to be living with AIDS (40 percent), and the greatest proportion of people who died with AIDS (50 percent).[18] Five of the ten states reporting the largest number of AIDS cases were in the South (Florida, Texas,

Georgia, Maryland, and North Carolina), and seven of the ten states reporting the highest rate of AIDS cases were in the South (Washington, D.C., Maryland, Florida, Louisiana, Delaware, Georgia, and South Carolina).[19] This, too, was not a new phenomenon: the South had led the country in estimated number of adults and adolescents living with AIDS since 1993, and, from the beginning of the epidemic until 2006, the South led the nation in the estimated number of deaths from AIDS (197,209, or 36 percent).[20]

The demographics of HIV/AIDS across the South echoed the racially disproportionate shape of the epidemic in North Carolina. In the South, 55 percent of the estimated number of people living with AIDS were black. This fact actually reflected the larger reality of HIV in the United States: AIDS disproportionately affected African Americans, and African Americans disproportionately lived in the South. In 2007, African Americans accounted for 51 percent of the new HIV/AIDS diagnoses and 48 percent of those living with HIV/AIDS in the states reporting that information.[21] Since at least 1985, AIDS had a disproportionate impact on black communities, and by 1993 African Americans had actually surpassed Caucasians in terms of AIDS caseload in the country, despite making up less than 15 percent of the population.[22] In 2007, AIDS diagnosis rates for African Americans were ten times higher than for Caucasians (seven times higher for black men and twenty-two times higher for black women).[23]

The interrelated models on which I based my view of AIDS made little room for an AIDS epidemic that, from very early on, had disproportionately affected African Americans in the southern United States. They also left me ill prepared to explain to my students the reasons that African Americans were at greater risk for HIV in North Carolina. Perhaps I should not have been surprised: all societies frame diseases in complex ways, and these constructions have important consequences for how individuals and groups understand themselves in relation to those diseases and how communities and policymakers respond to those understandings.[24] A growing number of observers point out the "crisis of representation" that AIDS posed for African American communities in the late twentieth and early twenty-first centuries, namely that while HIV/AIDS disproportionately affected African Americans in those years, representations of the disease failed to reflect that reality.[25] My "quick and dirty" research also indicated that the American South suffered from a crisis of representation when it came to AIDS.

The mischaracterization of the AIDS epidemic was not an inconsequential oversight. Historians, policymakers, AIDS activists, and health professionals had largely directed their attention to other foci of the epidemic while southern AIDS went unaddressed. This was reflected in federal funding: despite the disproportionate burden of HIV/AIDS on the American South, southern states were receiving less federal dollars per case for HIV/AIDS care or prevention than the nation as a whole ($5,184/AIDS case versus $5,625/AIDS case for care and $1,579/AIDS case versus $1,766/AIDS case for prevention in 2001).[26] It was also reflected in the science: a literature review conducted in 2000 found that while African Americans had increasingly been affected by HIV/AIDS over time, less than 1 percent of the AIDS-related medical literature published between 1980 and 1999 explicitly addressed the epidemic in African American communities.[27] At least when it came to prevention, it was unclear whether the most culturally competent evidence was being applied to the affected communities.

The disproportionate impact of AIDS on African Americans and the American South had not gone entirely unnoticed, however. A few books did touch on AIDS in the South. Abraham Verghese's *My Own Country*, published in 1994, recounted his experience as an East Indian physician fighting AIDS in the mountains of eastern Tennessee.[28] Seeing a surprising amount of HIV in his small community, Verghese mapped the successive waves of viral transmission into and within his community and developed powerful insight into the reality of stigma in rural America. Kathryn Whetten-Goldstein and Trang Quyen Nguyen's *"You're the First One I've Told,"* published in 2003, also addressed the problem of AIDS in the South, looking specifically at the experiences of twenty-five people with AIDS to demonstrate the unique life courses and needs that members of the "second wave" of the HIV/AIDS epidemic brought to the health care system.[29] Whetten-Goldstein and Nguyen's work explored reasons that individual patients deprioritized HIV in their lives and recommended steps health care leaders could take to help those patients reprioritize the disease and obtain better care. Both books provided rich insight into the lives of people with AIDS in the South, but neither book endeavored to explain the means by which HIV/AIDS came disproportionately to affect African Americans (Whetten-Goldstein does make note of the fact, while Verghese largely leaves it unaddressed).

Other monographs explored the problem of AIDS among African Americans. Perhaps the best example is Cathy Cohen's *The Boundaries of Blackness* (1999), which explored the forces working within and upon African American communities that structured their responses to HIV/AIDS.[30] Cohen situated the experience of many African Americans within the black community's self-identity and socioeconomic context and posited HIV as one of many "cross cutting" issues faced by traditional black leaders. Black political leaders failed adequately to respond to HIV/AIDS, Cohen argued, for three reasons: first, those most often afflicted with the disease challenged the norms and values of conservative black institutions; second, these institutions identified which community needs counted as legitimate and therefore worthy of community support; and, finally, these institutions failed to connect other factors—like class, gender, and sexual orientation—to their linked-fate definition of racial or community identity. In this regard, the response of black leaders mirrored larger patterns of cultural marginalization affecting African American communities. Cohen's book is perhaps the most insightful one available for understanding the ability (or inability) of black groups to mobilize around AIDS, but Cohen's focus is on national black organizations and AIDS organizers and does not address the South specifically.

Jacob Levenson's book *The Secret Epidemic* (2004) did perhaps the best job linking AIDS in minority communities to AIDS in the American South.[31] In his book Levenson concludes that AIDS in black America occurred at the intersection of race, "civil rights, drug abuse, policing, religion, politics, public health, housing, . . . sexuality, sin, and virtue," locating the heart of the "black and white failure to stop" the epidemic's spread in America's "unbridgeable racial chasm."[32] The strength of Levenson's book is his attention to research on sociostructural influences on community risk. His writing drew me to the research of Roderick Wallace, Mindy Fullilove, Robert Fullilove, Adaora Adimora, James Thomas, and Sevgi Aral.[33] These researchers—many of whom are social epidemiologists—explored the influence that poverty, migration, segregation, STD rates, incarceration, sexual concurrency, and demographic instability had on infectious diseases. Their research prompted a question for me: to what extent could social epidemiology help me explain high rates of HIV at historically black colleges in rural North Carolina?

NORTH CAROLINA IS PERTINENT to the story of AIDS in America for several reasons. First, pathbreaking biomedical research was taking place in the state during the 1980s and 1990s. Researchers at the Burroughs Wellcome headquarters in North Carolina pioneered the first anti-HIV drug in 1986. Second, that same year, the U.S. Justice Department leveled its first AIDS discrimination penalties against a North Carolina hospital, and the United States Agency for International Development (USAID) launched its first international AIDS prevention program by contracting with North Carolina–based Family Health International. Third, North Carolina figured prominently in debates over AIDS policy. In 1986, the state's conservative U.S. senator Jesse Helms fired the first volley in what would become a decade-and-a-half-long fight against exceptionalist AIDS policies. Finally, North Carolina boasted a broad cross section of American culture: it provided a fascinating mix of rich and poor; urban and rural; black and white; straight and gay; liberal and conservative; New South and Old South; southerner and northerner; agriculture and industry; mountain, coastal, and heartland. The particularities of North Carolina's AIDS story foreground aspects of the disease that were often overlooked in more conventional narratives of the epidemic in New York or San Francisco. Still, North Carolina's experience is not entirely dissimilar from the experience of AIDS in the American South and across the country. Therefore, North Carolina's story is not only valuable for its own sake, but it resonates with the stories of other communities in the periphery and provides a more complete understanding of the experience of AIDS in America.

The work of the aforementioned scholars generated the key questions I sought to explore in my study. The first set of questions was why HIV had followed two different trajectories within North Carolina's black and white populations. What were the individual behavioral risk factors that put North Carolinians at risk for HIV acquisition? Had those behaviors changed over time? And what—if anything—made those behaviors more common or more risky for African Americans in the state? Beyond HIV's underlying etiology and modes of transmission (which were well known), how did sociostructural forces like patterns of risk, race relations, gender relations, sexual identity, socioeconomic status, and living conditions in North Carolina influence HIV transmission among individuals and groups? In particular, were there sociostructural forces that left some groups more vulnerable to HIV transmission and infection than others in North Carolina, and if so, what influence had they had on North Carolina's AIDS epidemic?

The second set of questions I sought to answer related to policy and interventions; namely, what HIV care, treatment, and prevention strategies had North Carolinians developed to address HIV, and how effective had those efforts been. I knew from my exposure to Ronald Bayer's work that HIV had been approached differently from other public health problems, but what actual impact did AIDS exceptionalism have on HIV rates? What public health tradeoffs were involved in such strategies? And how uniform was the application of AIDS exceptionalist policies in states like North Carolina? Moreover, I was interested in finding out what effect a patient-initiated prevention strategy like VCT might have on different population groups (whether gay or straight, black or white, drug-using or not) and whether different levels of individual and population vulnerability might limit the effectiveness of such a strategy.

The answers to these questions, I hoped, would not only tell me something about HIV in North Carolina in the early twenty-first century but also offer insight into the larger shape of the epidemic in the American South and the greater United States. I hoped they would illuminate the extent to which HIV strategies from the "metropole" influenced efforts in more peripheral places like North Carolina and the whether those strategies adequately addressed the contours of North Carolina's epidemic. In the end, I also hoped it would help explain racial HIV disparities in the state, the South, and across the nation. This, in turn, might give me some sort of satisfactory answer to provide my students.

MUCH OF THE PRIMARY SOURCE material for this book comes from oral histories I conducted between 2006 and 2010. I have drawn from oral history collections, as well, most prominently from the work of historian Ian Lekus, who conducted interviews with many of North Carolina's earliest AIDS advocates, and have consulted similar sources located at Duke University, the University of North Carolina at Chapel Hill, as well as records from local media organizations. The internal documents of AIDS organizations in North Carolina were either shared with me by members of those organizations, or stored in the Lesbian and Gay Health Project (LGHP) archives at Duke University. The LGHP archives are a particularly rich source of material for the internal life of AIDS organizations in North Carolina, and their comprehensive nature owes a great deal to the hard work of LGHP members and Ian Lekus. The fact that each of the aforementioned sources centers on or springs from the Raleigh-Durham region of the Triangle clearly flavors this study, but I nonetheless believe the findings are relatively fair to the available data. The statistical data comes from official CDC or North Carolina sources, though in some cases the various analyses are from more comprehensive unpublished reports provided to me by government staff. I have also drawn on newspaper and medical literature in the public record. In this case, it should be noted, the data is skewed toward larger cities in the state, which have more robust media resources than smaller communities.

I should also make some preliminary statements about some of the terms used in this study. One of the phrases I employ repeatedly is "men who have sex with men," or MSM. Researchers have come to use this phrase because not all men who have sex with men consider themselves gay or bisexual, and many more have chosen not to identify themselves as such. The term "gay" signifies a socially constructed identity rather than a set of behaviors, and it does not encapsulate the totality of all men who have sex with men. A related term I employ is "communities." It is often tempting in both academic and public parlance to group individuals into larger social networks and to label those networks "communities." Methodological ease often trumps accuracy when those groups are defined (internally or externally) by such organizing factors as race, class, gender, or sexual behavior. Categories like "gay" or "African American" are socially constructed terms that can obfuscate differences within groups as much as they can clarify commonalities. Consequently, I have frequently opted to discuss "communities" rather than "the [insert term] community" to suggest that "communities" are heterogeneous and that members of various subpopulations do not all share the same level of HIV risk.

Additionally, one of the key issues I raise involves the policy debates around HIV testing. In North Carolina, the key policy debate hinged on whether HIV testing should be "anonymous" or "confidential" (also called "name-based", particularly in relation to contact-tracing procedures used by public health practitioners). I use the terms "confidential" and "name-based" interchangeably, and they stand in opposition to anonymous testing. Except where otherwise noted, however, both proponents of "anonymous" testing and those of "confidential" testing largely presume patient-initiated, voluntary counseling and testing.

Finally, throughout this work I make frequent reference to "social conservatives." By this I mean those individuals and groups that embrace similar, frequently "traditionalist," values relating to civil liberties, social relations, and sexual and reproductive freedoms, and who seek to preserve those values in modern society through public adherence and civil regulation.[34] While communities that adhere to these values have heterogeneous sociodemographic characteristics, I have generally avoided trying to describe them largely because analyzing the constitution of those groups is beyond the scope of this study. Instead I describe particular positions that would be deemed "socially conservative" and then label supporters of those positions "social conservatives."[35] That said, however, when those positions take concrete political manifestation, such as in the form of legislation, regulation, or curriculum, I describe the key actors in those efforts by name or position. Since social conservatism crosses political party, I tried not to conflate party affiliation with adherence to socially conservative norms.

The shape of this book is relatively straightforward. In chapter 1, I explore the earliest cases of AIDS in the state of North Carolina, some factors that could have amplified viral transmission in the state, and the relative abilities vulnerable groups had to organize against the epidemic once it emerged.

I trace the formation of North Carolina's first AIDS Service Organization among gay men, the Lesbian and Gay Health Organization (LGHP), and explore the values, interests, and concerns that shaped its care and prevention strategies. I also explore why other affected groups proved unable to launch similar movements at this time. In chapter 2, I continue my discussion of the LGHP, paying particular attention to the shape of its services, the role it played in the launch of AIDS groups in other cities, and the alliances its leaders develop with state health workers to promote noncoercive AIDS policies in a relatively conservative state. In chapter 3, I turn to efforts within the African American community to respond to AIDS and the various factors that shaped what that response looked like. I also trace the role that white gay men played in defining AIDS policy in North Carolina at the end of the 1980s. Chapter 4 investigates the transformation of HIV/AIDS that began in the late 1980s and early 1990s as improved therapies suggested HIV infection could become a chronic disease. I focus on the way the transformation began eroding the policy alliance that AIDS activists had developed with health officials and the consequences these changes had on state AIDS policy. I also examine the factors that facilitated HIV's unhindered spread into black communities during these years. Chapter 5 chronicles the further collapse of the alliance gay activists had built with health professionals and the consequences this had on North Carolina's HIV testing and surveillance policies. It also analyzes the factors that permitted HIV to seep deeply into the social networks of urban and rural blacks and the consequences this had on the shape of the epidemic in North Carolina by the mid-1990s. Finally, chapter 6 provides a snapshot of the AIDS epidemic in North Carolina in the latter half of the 1990s, paying particular attention to the state's care, treatment, and prevention policies in these years and the role those policies played in greater HIV acquisition and poorer HIV outcomes among African Americans. I also discuss the way that these trends in North Carolina were echoed across the South and the various efforts health workers made to address them. In my conclusion, I return to the questions my students asked me and some of the answers this study suggests. I also offer some suggestions about what this research might tell us about HIV in the American South and the greater United States.

CHAPTER 1

AIDS AND THE FRIGHTENING FUTURE
The Emergence of AIDS in North Carolina

In March 1983, Glenn Rowand discovered a small, pimple-sized purple spot on his arm. Over the next month, the physician's assistant watched the spot grow at an alarming rate. On May 9, physicians at Duke University Medical Center confirmed Rowand's fears: the unusual, purple spot on his arm was Kaposi's sarcoma; forty-seven-year-old Glenn Rowand had AIDS.[1]

While tragic in its own right, Rowand's diagnosis would play an important role in the history of North Carolina's fight against AIDS. Rowand had figured actively in the Triangle's gay life since the early 1970s.[2] A self-described "stereotypical AIDS victim," Rowand estimated having "in excess of 3,000 sexual contacts" in the period before his diagnosis, along with frequent butyl nitrate use and a long list of sexually transmitted diseases.[3] In the weeks and months that followed, Rowand and his partner, Douglas Ruhren, negotiated what journalist Sue Anne Pressley called the "frightening future" of his disease: they contacted former partners, adopted celibacy, changed jobs, and weathered Rowand's physical collapse.[4] Uncertain of how long he had left to live, Rowand decided to devote his remaining time educating other gay men about how to avoid AIDS. The education and support network that grew up around Glenn Rowand would come to define the shape of North Carolina's AIDS care and prevention policy over the next decade.

In many ways, the response in North Carolina to cases like that of Glenn Rowand mirrors the response to AIDS by gay men in countless other states. Influenced by local cases and the growing national concern over HIV, white gays and their allies in North Carolina took the initiative in caring for fellow gay men stricken with the disease—particularly those who had been abandoned by their families. These initially ad hoc responses eventually formalized in ways that came to shape statewide AIDS policies. For our purposes, what is important about Glenn Rowand's response to his illness—deciding to help educate others about AIDS— is that similar efforts were not made among other at-risk groups. From the beginning of the epidemic in North

Carolina, African Americans were disproportionately affected by AIDS. Yet no "Glenn Rowand" figure emerged in the African American community around whom a network of concern could develop to meet the needs of black men and women with AIDS. This chapter explores the factors that put some members of the African American community at greater risk for HIV infection, as well as the obstacles that prevented an AIDS care and prevention program from emerging from within the community.

HIV/AIDS WAS RELATIVELY rare in North Carolina in the earliest years of the epidemic. The first official case surfaced in Chapel Hill in June 1981, after physicians diagnosed a New York man with *Pneumocystis carinii* pneumonia and cytomegalovirus.[5] More migrant cases soon emerged in Winston-Salem and Greensboro, and then in January 1982, Chapel Hill doctors diagnosed the state's first indigenous case.[6] By the end of 1983, at least sixteen men in the state had been diagnosed with HIV/AIDS, eleven of whom were indigenous to North Carolina.[7] Of those twelve men whose race was identified, five (42 percent) were African Americans. Glenn Rowand belonged to a very small population of star-crossed men in those early years.

Such low numbers meant that other parts of the country properly drew greater attention in terms of AIDS response policy. But these low numbers should not be confused with low risk levels: several factors put North Carolina at risk for rapid viral spread as the epidemic unfolded. First, recent migration into the state put North Carolina at long-term risk for viral spread. North Carolina had seen substantial in-migration during the 1970s, reversing five decades of outmigration (fig. 1.1).[8] Troubled labor markets in New York, Florida, and California drew thousands of migrants to the new jobs in North Carolina and across the New South.[9] Most of these migrants moved to cities like Charlotte, Raleigh, and Greensboro, and some, unwittingly, brought the virus with them.

Other forms of migration also served to bring HIV to the state: drug traffic, drug tourism, sex tourism, seasonal migration, and return migration. Since the completion of the national highways in the 1950s and 1960s, cities like Fayetteville and Durham became havens for drug traffic since North Carolina served as a midway point along the east coast drug route stretching from Florida to New York.[10] Many North Carolinians were also "drug tourists," using drugs while visiting other parts of the country and then returning home.[11] Others from the Tar Heel state (50 percent of gay respondents in at least one local survey) reported having sex with people "in large cities . . . such as Atlanta, Houston, New York, San Francisco, and Los Angeles" in

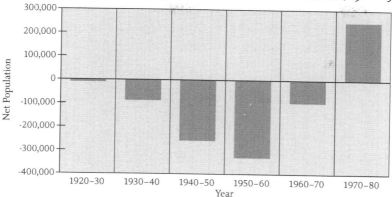

FIGURE 1.1. Net Population Migration to and from North Carolina, 1920–1980

Source: The North Carolina Atlas Revisited, http://www.ncatlasrevisited.org/homefrm.html.

the early 1980s.[12] Additionally, some North Carolina counties saw upwards of two thousand seasonal workers travel through their borders each year, as thousands of farmers across the state relied on seasonal labor to harvest hundreds of thousands of acres of cultivated land.[13] Finally, many people with AIDS returned to North Carolina to receive care from their families; between 1981 and 1983, for example, 55 percent of the individuals with AIDS in North Carolina came from New York or Florida.[14] All of these forms of migration served as a possible means by which HIV entered the state.[15]

Once in North Carolina, HIV had several environments in which to flourish. Long-term, concentrated poverty and unemployment rendered certain communities extremely vulnerable to HIV infection when it arrived. A key problem for poor people—especially women and minorities—was their diminished access to medical care.[16] Inferior access to timely medical care permitted valuable time to pass before physicians could diagnose and treat an individual's health problems, leaving poor people and minorities with diminished overall health and greater vulnerabilities to HIV when it entered their communities.[17] Impoverished communities also suffer HIV-facilitating problems, including elevated sexually transmitted infection (STI) rates, increased drug marketing, and heightened social disorganization.[18]

Other factors beyond poverty rendered North Carolina communities vulnerable to HIV transmission. The presence of STIs provides one example. STIs can amplify the transmissibility of HIV (herpes simplex 2, for example, increases the transmissibility of HIV by two to four times), so a heightened prevalence of STIs in a given population would place it at greater risk for HIV infection and transmission.[19] In the first half of the 1980s, North Carolina's syphilis rates equaled the national average, gonorrhea rates stood twice as high, and gay men and minorities reported rates even higher.[20] Concurrent sexual partnerships serve as another example. If even a small number of individuals within a sexual network change partners frequently, STIs can transmit dramatically in a given population; indeed, the more partners individuals have, the faster and greater will be that spread.[21] In North Carolina in the early 1980s, surveys indicated that upwards of 52 percent of gay men had more than one sexual partner each month, and later research suggested that between one-quarter and one-half of minorities reported at least one instance in which they had concurrent sexual relationships in the previous five years.[22] Since these sexual networks entailed relatively modest sized groupings, a malicious virus could wreak extensive damage in a relatively short period of time.[23] Consequently the rates of sexually transmitted infections, the frequency of sexual concurrence, and the relatively constricted size of the sexual networks put several communities in North Carolina at risk for HIV infection. All of these factors, it turns out, would weigh heavily in the spread of HIV in North Carolina, and they would affect African Americans in a particularly deleterious fashion.

WHILE HIV THREATENED a variety of subpopulations in North Carolina, members of the state's white gay communities responded first to the challenge of HIV/AIDS. Gays were able to do this not only because HIV uniquely affected their communities but also because local gay and lesbian communities already boasted several sophisticated activists, possessed extensive organization and networking skills, and exhibited incipient organizing around gay and lesbian health concerns. As elsewhere, North Carolina's HIV epidemic disproportionately affected gay Caucasian men. In the first three years of the state's epidemic, about 60 percent of the cases occurred among Caucasian men; where exposure categories were reported, every one of these cases occurred among men who had sex with men (MSM).[24] The disease, then, concentrated in a specifically beleaguered minority community.

The disease took hold in a community that, since the 1970s, had become particularly mobilized to exert their civil liberties in the face of often fierce local and national discrimination.[25] Gay men and lesbians in North Carolina faced hate crimes and prejudice locally, while their national representatives—particularly Senator Jesse Helms—waged a national effort against gay equality. In response, gays and lesbians in North Carolina generated a robust rights movement: They opened social venues, founded student groups, launched media outlets, and created affirming cultural events.[26] By 1980, even black lesbians and gays had founded their own groups (called UMOJA, which means "unity" in Swahili), although black gays still remained considerably more concealed than their white counterparts. Consequently, lesbians and gays established growing political clout in the state, leading to antidiscrimination laws in cities like Chapel Hill and gay rights marches in places like Durham.

The desire for autonomy and nondiscrimination in sexual matters easily translated into expectations for autonomy and nondiscrimination in larger health-related matters. Inspired by the women's health movement and motivated by local experiences of discrimination, gay activists in Durham began organizing a gay and lesbian health organization in the fall of 1982,[27] drawing on local social networks to build their movement.[28] One of the activists— nationally renowned Carl Wittman—felt the best way gay men and lesbians could handle medical intolerance was through the formation of alternative sources of care: culturally competent clinics where gays and lesbians could care for one another in an oppression-free environment. Another budding activist, public health student David Jolly, hoped to establish a referral service so that local gays and lesbians could find culturally competent clinicians and an education program to train culturally competent health practitioners to ensure that lesbians and gays received adequate health care delivery. With these visions in mind, Wittman, Jolly, and two lesbian friends—Timmer McBride and Aida Wakil—met on a cool evening in November 1982 to launch the Lesbian and Gay Health Project (LGHP).[29] It would quickly become North Carolina's first AIDS Service Organization.

Even before AIDS had been named and identified as a problem for gays, the need for such an organization seemed obvious. Both lesbians and gay men complained of receiving suboptimal care from health providers. "The health needs of our community are not being met," the four would later write; gays and lesbians frequently suffered "overt discrimination, insensitivity to their concerns, and ignorance of [their] problems."[30] Many worried "about the social, economic, and legal consequences of [their] sexual preferences being discovered."[31] "We must be our own advocates," they concluded, " . . . our health care needs will not be met unless we are active in defining those needs and implementing the services to meet them."[32] Cofounder Carl Wittman— an acclaimed antiwar and gay rights activist who wrote for Students for a Democratic Society before penning the 1969 gay declaration, "Refugees from Amerika: A Gay Manifesto"—favored an entirely indigenous effort: lesbians and gays controlling their own medical care.[33] Wakil, McBride, and Jolly envisioned a more hybridized approach: the group would advocate for nondiscriminatory health care in mainstream settings while working to establish alternative health care for gay men and lesbians across the state.[34] They would draw attention to gay and lesbian health issues, exert their rights to quality health care, and demand those rights and expectations from their health care providers.[35] To accomplish its goals, the group would conduct a needs survey, launch a "health information and referral" program based on their findings, create a health support network for gays and lesbians, and eventually open lesbian and gay health clinics throughout the state.[36]

Meanwhile, the AIDS threat percolated just below the surface for Jolly and Wittman. Both men had already heard about the new disease, and the news terrified them. "I had heard about [AIDS] that summer [of 1982]," Jolly recalled in an interview. "It was the first time I remember hearing about it. . . . I think it would have probably been through the gay press, because my straight friends hadn't heard anything about it at that point. We were terrified. . . . None of us knew whether we were going to get it, so for me it was like, 'I don't need these daily reminders of my vulnerability thank you very much.'"[37] With many gay contacts across the country, Wittman had likewise learned of the disease. As local news coverage of AIDS increased at the end of 1982 and into 1983, Jolly and Wittman began to plan how they might respond to the problem: coordinating local treatments, educating local doctors, mobilizing local gays to respond.[38] With local concern growing, Jolly and Wittman began compiling articles on the problem, planning a seminar with the latest information on the epidemic, and preparing a potential support program for people who got sick.[39] They still knew no one locally with the disease, however.

AIDS AFFECTED OTHER GROUPS in North Carolina besides gay men: hemophiliacs, blood product recipients, injection drug users, and certain African Americans also bore the brunt of the epidemic. But while each of these groups possessed the leadership potential and resource networks adequate to respond to the situation, only gay men and their allies mounted an organized response to the disease in those early years. Americans have come to expect interest groups to mobilize in response to various health issues, but in this case, the other affected groups lacked decisive factors critical to effective mobilization on AIDS.[40]

Hemophiliacs were well positioned to organize on AIDS once the threat became clear because they had a strong network of support linked through the local Hemophilia Treatment Center at the University of North Carolina's Comprehensive Hemophilia Diagnostic and Treatment Center; they shared a collective identity around similar life experiences; and they had a strong national organization, the National Hemophilia Foundation, advocating on their behalf.[41] However, several factors worked against a strong activist role by hemophiliacs in the state: the at-risk population was small (540 hemophiliacs lived in the state) and young (most were boys); no hemophiliacs in the state received an AIDS diagnosis in the first half of the 1980s; and hemophiliac families had a symbiotic relationship with medical professionals.[42] Hemophiliacs lacked the proper positioning to play a major role in North Carolina's AIDS-advocacy movement.[43] People in North Carolina became exposed to HIV-infected blood or tissue as early as 1982, but blood transfusion/tissue transplant recipients had few collective bonds, which made them even less likely to organize for health advocacy.[44]

For their part, substance abusers had access to a string of addiction resources across the state from which a robust anti-AIDS campaign could have come. But while one-fifth of the state's early AIDS cases occurred among injection drug users, addicts appeared unaware of the problem. As a thirty-four-year-old former addict told reporters in the summer of 1983, "I would suspect they'd only be concerned if they came down with [AIDS] . . . . I don't think they have time to be concerned. They're busy getting and using drugs." And state addiction specialists agreed (according to the head of one Charlotte clinic, "the active needle user . . . is probably not very concerned about health problems") and considered infectious disease control to be outside their purview.[45]

African Americans also had a rich tradition of community action in North Carolina on which to build an anti-AIDS movement. A robust response to AIDS failed to materialize, however, for several reasons. First, the earliest African American cases appeared among different risk groups at different hospitals in different counties across the state. Second, black men with AIDS died much more quickly after diagnosis than their white counterparts.[46] Third, few black men served as health activists or health care professionals in the state. Fourth, reports of AIDS among African Americans were often delayed getting to the Centers for Disease Control and Prevention (CDC) and absent in the media. Fifth, black gay groups lacked the power to make AIDS an issue, while local and national African American interest groups focused their attention on more pervasive socioeconomic concerns.[47] Consequently, AIDS did not directly align with the shared racial identity of these men; their more rapid demise may have prevented their loved ones from connecting individual illnesses to larger trends; too few people in positions of knowledge could recognize a collective threat or generate a collective response on their behalf; and no local or national black groups compensated for this absence.[48] It would be some time before AIDS activism emerged within North Carolina's black communities. In North Carolina, then, only gay men became deeply engaged with AIDS in these early years. Such a lopsided response played an important role in the shape of the epidemic as it unfolded in North Carolina.

WHILE GAY MEN WERE WELL POSITIONED to respond to HIV/AIDS in North Carolina, an organized response was not automatic. Most of the program planning fell to David Jolly. The Princeton graduate hailed from Connecticut, but he spent most of the 1970s teaching elementary school in Boston. In 1980, Jolly enrolled in the University of North Carolina's School of Public Health to obtain a master's degree in Health Policy and Administration, and in 1982, he began pursuing his doctorate in public health. As the group's public health expert, Jolly began looking for response resources outside the state. In the spring of 1983, Jolly learned that activists planned to hold the second national forum on AIDS at June's National Lesbian and Gay Health Conference (NLGHC) in Denver. The conference would offer Jolly the chance to tap into the larger lesbian and gay health movement while providing him insight into early responses to AIDS, so in June he traveled to Denver to attend the forum.[49]

The NLGHC, which was launched in 1978 to promote health care equality for gays and lesbians, helped shape early national AIDS policy. At the 1982 conference, some participants discussed the emerging, but still unnamed, epidemic among gay men. By 1983, more was known about the syndrome, and representatives from leading AIDS groups—including Gay Men's Health Crisis (New York), the KS Research and Education Foundation (San Francisco), and the AIDS Project Los Angeles—met to share care, treatment, and prevention strategies.[50] AIDS was becoming a highly contentious issue across the country in the summer of 1983. San Francisco was debating bathhouse regulations; hospitals were debating infection-control measures to protect health workers; and federal officials clashed with gay activists and blood industry executives over testing blood and screening donors.[51] While the NLGHC activists disagreed about which safer sex guidelines to back, they opposed donor screening, blood quarantining, bathhouse restrictions, and any attempts to moralize the epidemic.[52] Standard, coercive strategies of mainstream public health would be unacceptable and ineffective, they concluded; the risk of AIDS should not threaten gay men's collective rights or individual liberties.[53]

Armed with the resources gleaned from the "amazing . . . [and] life altering" conference, Jolly returned to North Carolina excited to begin working on gay and lesbian health and desperate to start something on AIDS.[54] But since Jolly still knew no one in North Carolina with AIDS, he did not foresee AIDS becoming a large part of LGHP's task list very quickly. That changed soon after his return, however, when he received a call from Glenn Rowand.

In the month since his diagnosis, Rowand changed his life dramatically. He stopped having sex with his partner and other men; he stopped cooking for friends out of fear he might transmit his disease through the food; and he transferred out of direct patient care in his job at Duke University Medical Center. In the days after that initial diagnosis, he and his partner contacted forty of Rowand's most recent sexual contacts to inform them of his disease status. And this spirit of concern prompted the men to contact David Jolly in mid-June 1983, to see whether Jolly's Lesbian and Gay Health Project could help them equip local men to prepare for AIDS.[55]

Glenn Rowand's personal experience catalyzed the AIDS effort in North Carolina. Jolly and the other LGHP founders immediately started meeting with Rowand to put a support team in place. By the end of June, six people had volunteered to help care for men with AIDS.[56] This spike in the number of volunteers proved prescient because Rowand's diagnosis had sparked a rush of AIDS concern among local men: many of Rowand's sexual contacts and acquaintances quickly scheduled appointments at Duke Hospital to ascertain their own AIDS status.[57] With Rowand's disclosure, the intermittent trickle of AIDS patients coming into Duke became a steady stream. Less than a month after Rowand's diagnosis, Duke launched a clinic for patients with AIDS. "We were seeing so many people who were concerned," explained Duke's chief of infectious diseases, Dr. David Durack, "that we decided the best thing to do was to have a clinic for patients."[58] Within weeks, almost fifty people had flocked to the clinic, twelve of whom showed symptoms associated with AIDS.[59] The stream of AIDS patients continued to grow into the fall of 1983, and the necessity for care and support came with them. AIDS quickly began to consume the Lesbian and Gay Health Project, and by the end of the year the volunteer staff decided to formalize their efforts around AIDS.

NORTH CAROLINA'S AFRICAN AMERICAN community failed to respond to AIDS in an organized way in these early years. AIDS struck too diverse and diffuse a group of black men too quickly to allow an AIDS response program to emerge. Adding to this, AIDS affected stigmatized and powerless sub-populations within black communities; those affected had few champions who could herald their cause in a way that would gain national recognition or sympathy, especially with the heavy weight of socioeconomic concerns already pressing on African American communities during the double-digit inflation and unemployment of the early 1980s.

This absence of advocates proved particularly noteworthy because AIDS disproportionately affected African Americans from the very beginning of the epidemic in North Carolina. As previously mentioned, 42 percent of the earliest cases occurred among African Americans.[60] Added to this was the fact that several biosocial factors portended greater risk for HIV transmission among African Americans in the state. Lacking advocates left many African Americans unaware of risk factors they might otherwise have avoided or against which they might have protected themselves.

THE STRUCTURE OF SEXUAL networks proved to be one of the most important biosocial factors that increased the risk of HIV transmission in North Carolina's African American community. In the early 1980s, gonorrhea rates were four times higher than the national average, and syphilis rates topped out at almost six times as high.[61] Since STIs can increase the transmissibility of HIV, many in the African American community were extremely vulnerable. Rates of infection were so pronounced among African Americans, in part, because sexual networks in North Carolina remained relatively bounded by race. While the era of formal segregation had ended by this time, white people still did not live in the same communities as black people, much less sleep with them. Since sexual networks in the state—both gay and straight—were segregated along racial lines, networks among minorities were smaller and more contained, meaning an individual within those networks was far more likely to have sexual contact with someone who had many sexual partners, regardless of his own number of partners.[62] Even African Americans in North Carolina who reported having very few sexual partners were five times more likely than whites and four times more likely than Hispanics to have a sexual partner who had had four or more sexual partners.[63]

Additionally, variables within sexual networks—like sex ratios and sexual concurrency—put African American communities at greater risk for HIV infection. Sex ratios (the ratio of males to females in a population) played an important role in sexual patterns and community stability. Epidemiologists Adimora and Schoenbach note that, in the United States, "black populations . . . have sustained the most severe and persistent shortage of men of any subculture since documentation by modern censuses."[64] In the 1980s, the sex ratio among African Americans in North Carolina fell to 0.88 (for black women between the ages of twenty-five and forty-four it was 0.86, and for women in their thirties it was 0.84).[65] Lower sex ratios led to lower marriage rates and higher divorce rates and put women at a disadvantage in terms of negotiating fidelity or the use of prophylaxis.[66] Low sex ratios and relational instability make it more likely men will have more sexual partners and less likely they will use condoms. Sexual concurrency also contributed to the spread of STIs; if a small number of individuals within a sexual network change partners frequently, the "transmission and persistence of a curable STI" within that population would be dramatic.[67] In North Carolina in the 1980s, studies suggested that one-quarter of black women and one-half of black men had engaged in at least one concurrent sexual relationship in the previous five years.[68]

These sexual networks were embedded in a larger sociostructural matrix that included issues of poverty, migration, health access, incarceration, unemployment, and community cohesion. Historically, diseases like HIV have disproportionately affected the poor because the poor live with inferior nutrition, limited health care, and riskier surroundings. In North Carolina in the early 1980s, African Americans bore the brunt of poverty and long-term joblessness in the state.[69] This translated into tremendous racially based economic disparities. During the recession in the 1980s (1981–83), North Carolina's unemployment rate topped out at over 10 percent, but African Americans suffered a rate over twice as high.[70] Consequently, African Americans carried a heavier burden of poverty; 30.4 percent of the state population and 33.2 percent of the population in eastern North Carolina (as opposed to 10 percent of whites across the state and 12.4 percent in eastern North Carolina).[71] Since poverty—especially long-term concentrated poverty and joblessness —generates problems that facilitate the spread of HIV in communities, including elevated STI rates, increased drug use, and heightened social disorganization, certain African American communities were extremely vulnerable to HIV infection when it arrived.[72]

In addition to poverty, migration put black communities at higher risk for HIV infection. After the Great Migration, African Americans began returning to North Carolina (and other parts of the South) en masse (see table 1.1).[73] Of particular significance, this "Great Return Migration" concentrated in southern cities, and it disproportionately involved black women. This meant that black women, some possibly with HIV, were returning to riskier locales (cities), where they further skewed the already low sex ratios of those communities.

On top of voluntary migration was the problem of forced migration, otherwise known as incarceration. Incarceration disproportionately affected

TABLE 1.1. Black Migration to and from North Carolina, 1965–1980

Period	North Carolina	Charlotte	Triangle	Triad	Fayetteville	Rocky Mount
1965–70	-29,732	121	-1,100	1,392	3,883	-3,145
1975–80	14,456	2,725	5,774	5,120	7,053	-1,368

Source: William H. Frey, "The New Great Migration: Black Americans' Return to the South, 1965–2000," in *The Brookings Institution, The Living Cities Census Series* (Washington, D.C.: The Brookings Institution, May 2004).

blacks: although they constituted only 20 percent of the state's population, they made up 55 percent of the prison population.[74] Research indicates that social control measures can often have unexpected consequences, and the "massive and concentrated" role of incarceration appears to have been an example of this in minority communities.[75] Research suggests that the mass incarceration of young men in minority communities created a macro-level "feedback loop that cause[d] disorganization." Incarceration may have lessened community liabilities, but it also "deplete[d] the community of assets" like family income and social support and stability (however modest those may have been). As Rose and Clear note, "At the ecological level, the side effects of policies intended to fight crime by controlling individual criminals may exacerbate problems that lead to crime in the first place."[76]

In terms of the spread of HIV in African American communities in North Carolina, incarceration policy played a pivotal role. Men or women who were left behind during their partners' incarceration and had depended financially on them frequently engaged in "separational concurrency" and "survival sex"; sex frequently became the most readily available exchange currency in these circumstances.[77] While in prison, inmates were often subjected to coercive sexual relationships with individuals at high risk for sexually transmitted infections.[78] If inmates joined gangs in prison, they became incorporated into new social networks that exposed them to risky sexual behavior, in addition to common prison behaviors like tattooing and injection drug use, which led to further potential exposure to viruses. Upon release, inmates often engaged in concurrent sexual relationships and continued to use drugs.

Finally, poor people's diminished access to medical care put them at greater risk for HIV transmission. North Carolina had relatively tough qualifying criteria for Medicaid, limiting the access of many uninsured people—especially women and minorities—to primary care (when compared to the access of those with private insurance).[79] Even where primary care proved accessible through Medicaid or employer-based insurance, many poor people in North Carolina postponed medical treatment owing to its costs, both in terms of time and out-of-pocket expenses.[80] In addition, many African Americans compounded these delays because they deeply distrusted the American health care system. Delays in access and timely treatment permitted valuable time to pass before physicians could diagnose and treat an individual's health problems.[81] Since, as Eileen Stillwaggon notes, poorer overall health ("[poor] nutrition, parasite load, and other diseases") rendered one's immune system more vulnerable to transmitting or acquiring HIV infection, inferior access to medical care left the poor and minorities more vulnerable to HIV when it entered their communities.[82]

AS I HAVE SHOWN, at the beginning of North Carolina's AIDS epidemic, subpopulations particularly vulnerable to HIV infection were unequally equipped to face the coming threat.[83] Injection drug users and transfusion recipients lacked the collective identity to mobilize around AIDS. Hemophiliacs were too integrated into the mainstream medical system, and many of their constituents were too young to develop an autonomous identity. African Americans, who suffered the most diverse expression of the epidemic, lacked both a local and national awareness of their own risk and faced a host of socioeconomic problems that dwarfed the emerging disease. Only white gay men in North Carolina sufficiently understood the epidemic's threat; only they had a strong, unified, and autonomous community equipped with the resources upon which to draw for an AIDS organization; and only they had insider access to medical professionals and health care resources that enabled them to create an infrastructure of care for people with AIDS.[84]

From the outset, then, the response to AIDS in North Carolina stood poised to adopt a very specific shape. White gay men and their allies in Durham, North Carolina, formed the Lesbian and Gay Health Project and began mobilizing against AIDS. It was one of fewer than fifty groups of its kind in the country.[85] Owing to the strength of the white gay community in North Carolina and the United States, the LGHP drew on preexisting resources at the local and national levels to fight AIDS, addressing concerns vital to gays and lesbians in the process. Privacy, one of the issues discussed by the activists in Denver, quickly became an important principle adopted by David Jolly and his LGHP colleagues in North Carolina.[86] Other groups affected by the epidemic may have offered alternative priorities in their approaches to fighting HIV/AIDS, but they failed to mobilize in North Carolina and would therefore lack a voice in AIDS policy development.[87]

CHAPTER 2

MAKING SURE THAT THIS TRAGEDY NEVER HAPPENS AGAIN

AIDS Organizing and North Carolina's Gay Community

O n a cold November day in Durham, North Carolina, a young Virginia man pulled into a parking space at Duke University Medical Center and made his way into the hospital. Months earlier, he had inexplicably started feeling tired and slightly depressed. Over the next months his fatigue worsened, he rapidly lost weight, his lymph nodes swelled, and he was unable to shake a persistent, low-grade fever. Eventually, the fear he had suppressed for so long broke the surface of his psyche: he had AIDS.

He lived in a southern Virginia town with his parents, where everyone knew everyone, and where everyone looked on gays with disgust. And he was gay. His parents remained oblivious to this fact, or at least he hoped they did. AIDS, however, would reveal the truth to his parents in the worst possible way. They would learn their son was both gay and dying, and he would face the double rejection of a "deplorable lifestyle" and a stigmatized disease.

He remained uncertain whether he actually had the virus, though, and so he headed south, hoping against hope as he crossed the Virginia border and sped through the rolling hills of North Carolina toward Duke University Medical Center that it was something else — anything else.

But it was there, in his room at Duke hospital on November 6, 1984, that the young man learned that indeed he did have Pneumocystis carinii pneumonia — a sure sign of AIDS. And it was there, in his bathroom at Duke hospital on November 6, 1984, that the young man cut his throat, slit his wrists, and died. It was hard enough being a gay man in the South; he had no desire also to be a person with AIDS.[1]

This young Virginia man represented the struggle in which members of the Lesbian and Gay Health Project (LGHP) found themselves. "Making sure that this tragedy never happens again is one of the purposes of the Durham-based Lesbian and Gay Health Project," wrote David Jolly, in the November 20 edition of North Carolina's gay newspaper the *Front Page*.[2] The support program that had grown up around Glenn Rowand pioneered AIDS care in North Carolina, but the needs of people caught up in the epidemic soon grew larger than the ad hoc group could handle. Consequently, the LGHP formalized its structure and extended its influence across the state. The shape this response took had important consequences for the contours of AIDS policy in the state in the ensuing years. This chapter traces the origins, development, and consequences of these policy decisions for North Carolina's AIDS epidemic.

ONE OF THE MOST IMMEDIATE concerns for Jolly and Wittman was awareness of local AIDS risk. Most gay men in the state felt little concern about AIDS: "Initially [AIDS] was a joke," noted one gay man from Chapel Hill.

> People didn't know what it was, and there were very few people who were diagnosed, and I think about being at a dinner party in . . . the early 80s . . . and this topic came up, and somebody was saying, "Well, I read an article in the paper that these people who have this disease were having up to fifty sexual partners a day." And I remember somebody laughing, and saying, "Oh! I am lucky that I only had forty-eight yesterday!" You know and it was that sort of thing. But people didn't— it was something that happened to a couple of people in San Francisco and New York.[3]

A gay bar patron in Charlotte concurred in the summer of 1983: "I think if I were living in a major metropolitan area—New York or San Francisco—I would personally have some concern. I'm not living my life worrying about whether I have AIDS. . . . There's not a lot I can do about it. If I choose to be celibate from this point out, it may be too late anyway."[4] Indeed, with no known cases, men in Charlotte felt little risk. "I don't think there's really a lot of concern in Charlotte," noted a bar manager. "It's more a subject to talk about. It's one of those things where a person says, 'Yeah, but this can't happen to me.' Though I wouldn't wish it on anybody, I hope someone comes across a documented case of AIDS. We need a good scare. The majority of people feel too smug that it can't happen here."[5]

Jolly and Wittman held few illusions about local vulnerabilities, however. Glenn Rowand's list of sexual partners painted a grim picture: at least forty locals had sex with him in the previous year alone. Each one represented an additional vector of infection. Moreover, results from Jolly and Wittman's Lesbian and Gay Health Survey began coming in, revealing just how risky were the sexual lives of local men. Few knew about AIDS, and most reported multiple anonymous partners—many from the epidemic's epicenters—and high rates of STIs.[6] Since by now most medical professionals suspected the source of AIDS to be an infectious agent, many locals stood at risk.

To raise awareness, Jolly and Wittman created a two-hour AIDS presentation for local gay organizations. The program included up-to-date AIDS information, explored the sociopolitics of the epidemic, and discussed the personal implications of the disease. Glenn Rowand frequently joined them to talk about life with AIDS. In the second half of 1983, Jolly and Wittman took their program to social clubs, religious groups, and academic organizations across the state.[7] They also wrote articles and gave media interviews on AIDS.[8] By the end of 1983, LGHP was a leading source for AIDS information in the state.

Equally important, particularly for Jolly, was AIDS care and support.[9] Glenn Rowand foreshadowed the problem: by mid-1983, AIDS cases in the state began climbing. Most of the first people with AIDS were those returning home from elsewhere to receive care from their families. Tony Adinolfi, an intensive care nurse at Duke and one of the LGHP's earliest volunteers, recalled that "in '83 we were getting kids from all over the country whose families lived in the Southeast, and they were really sick."[10] People came because, by 1983, Duke University Medical Center in Durham and UNC Medical Center in Chapel Hill had become hubs for AIDS care and research. Duke became an AIDS research magnet after Duke infectious disease specialist David Durack wrote the first editorial on AIDS for the *New England Journal of Medicine*.[11] The Medical Center opened a weekly AIDS clinic in May 1983 to address the ensuing influx of local and international AIDS patients.[12] At the same time, North Carolina Memorial Hospital in Chapel Hill saw most of the state's earliest AIDS cases and also treated many hemophiliacs with AIDS because it boasted the region's largest hemophilia treatment center.[13] Of course, doctors could offer patients little. "There was no drug," Tony Adinolfi remembered, "we would Fed-Ex pentamidine from the Centers for Disease Control and Prevention (CDC) back then. And that was the only drug we had to offer."[14] It was in this context of therapeutic helplessness that David Jolly and his LGHP volunteers began providing care and support for patients with AIDS.

Tony Adinolfi played a key role in this process. A gay man from the Northeast, Adinolfi had moved to Durham in May 1983 to work at the Veterans Hospital in Durham. His move coincided with the launch of the Health Project, so he became an early volunteer.[15] This connection proved fortuitous, because Adinolfi's role as house supervisor, evening supervisor, and ICU nurse at the Veterans Hospital gave him close contact with most of the active AIDS cases cycling through Durham at the time. "I took care of the really sick guys," he explained in an interview, "and then when they were transferred to the floor I would visit them. And that's how [the LGHP AIDS program] started, just the informal visitation."[16]

The "informal visits" gained structure in the fall of 1983 after Adinolfi encountered Mike Waycaster at Durham Veterans Hospital. Waycaster hailed from San Francisco but came to Durham to receive AIDS care closer to his western North Carolina family. While living in San Francisco, Waycaster had worked with a residential care program known as the Shanti Project, which cared for the terminally ill and in the early 1980s became one of the nation's leading AIDS organizations.[17] While in Durham, Waycaster taught Shanti's care model to the LGHP team (Waycaster initially commuted to Durham from western North Carolina for care but soon relocated to an apartment the Health Project found him near the hospital).[18] "[Waycaster] was endlessly patient," Jolly recalled. "So we started out by providing support services to Michael."[19] Since the VA lacked many amenities available at other hospitals, LGHP volunteers supplied them. "If you get a sore throat and you are in a regular hospital," explained Tony Adinolfi, "there's a [pediatrics] ward [where] they can get you a popsicle. The VA doesn't have anything like that. So that's what his buddies did."[20] The group also supplied moral support to Waycaster, because like many early patients with AIDS, Waycaster routinely found himself shunned by hospital staff.

Health officials offered conflicting messages regarding AIDS in 1983: some officials maintained that "there was no risk [of AIDS] from casual contact," while researchers suggested "the possibility that routine close contact, as within a family household, can spread the disease."[21] Opting (or panicking) for caution, many hospital staff viewed people with AIDS with fear and treated AIDS as a highly contagious disease.[22] Not infrequently, these concerns translated to discrimination and homophobia. In Michael Waycaster's case, for example, VA staff "wouldn't bring [his] food in. [They] left it outside his door. They'd come in moon suits to empty his trash."[23] Jolly, Adinolfi, and other LGHP volunteers compensated for this gap in care: until he died, they visited Waycaster in the hospital, brought him food, brushed his hair, cleaned his apartment, and hosted his family when they came to visit.[24]

LGHP volunteers also borrowed from other care models across the country, particularly the buddy model championed by the Gay Men's Health Crisis in

New York. Adinolfi would scout patients with AIDS through contacts at local hospitals and match them with at least one "buddy." Buddies became advocates and caregivers: they ensured that patients received appropriate care in the hospital and coordinated other support once the patient was discharged. "We forced ourselves in," Adinolfi explained. "[We went to local hospitals and] said, 'We've devised this buddy program based on Gay Men's Health Crisis that we would like you to take advantage of.'"[25] Hospitals were "very receptive." At Duke, for example, Adinolfi met regularly with the infectious disease staff to hear if they had any new patients with AIDS. "The doctors at Duke and the VA told me about people," explained Adinolfi. "I was the main person they told because I was right there. I was able to visit people and ask if they wanted our services. It was really a total violation of confidentiality, but there was nothing else, there was no other option."[26] LGHP volunteers offered similar services to the clinicians at North Carolina Memorial Hospital.[27]

The profoundly stigmatizing nature of AIDS in these early years made this support essential. For many of those infected with HIV, an AIDS diagnosis exposed their homosexuality to their unsuspecting family members, who in turn often responded with a combination of revulsion and terror. When families visited patients, many "refused to touch" their sons, opting instead to sit "across the room."[28] Some of those diagnosed with AIDS lacked the psychological wherewithal to handle such weighty news, and not an insignificant number committed suicide upon hearing their prognosis.[29] Others suffering from rejection from their family and friends might have lived their last days in isolation had not a LGHP volunteer visited them each day.[30] At the start of 1984, however, physicians had diagnosed sixteen people with AIDS in at least twelve counties across the state.[31] The spread of the disease in the state was quickly outstripping the LGHP's ability to provide ad hoc services and support.[32]

By the spring of 1984, with over sixty people with AIDS in eighteen counties in North Carolina, the LGHP began formalizing its growing AIDS services in the face of an accelerating epidemic. They upgraded their patient support program, AIDS awareness efforts, and volunteer training and recruitment plan throughout the year. This early in the epidemic, the LGHP became a key informant on the disease throughout the state. With so many people looking to the LGHP for AIDS information, Tony Adinolfi joined David Jolly giving seminars across the state and the greater southeast.[33] The group also upgraded and reprinted their information brochure, "AIDS: What You Should Know . . .," which it distributed throughout the state.[34]

LGHP's support system remained ad hoc, however, because the group lacked an organized means of reaching people with AIDS. Adinolfi and his colleagues learned of people with AIDS only through "personal contacts and word of mouth."[35] LGHP volunteers were therefore providing support for ten of North Carolina's sixty people with AIDS.[36] Consequently, many who might have benefited from LGHP services received limited support due to their personal isolation, their distance from the Triangle, or their lack of connection to white gay communities.[37] In June 1984, LGHP's steering committee recognized that the AIDS program could maximize its outreach to people with AIDS if it collaborated with North Carolina's epidemiology department to identify patients in need of care. Accordingly, it encouraged David Jolly to pursue any leads in that regard.[38]

Thus far in the epidemic, North Carolina's health department felt compelled to take an aggressive stance on AIDS. Public health institutions and state hospitals led by providing acute care for people with AIDS.[39] Additionally, beginning in April 1983, North Carolina's Medicaid program began providing limited support to people with AIDS after the federal Social Security Administration added AIDS to its list of recognized impairments covered by Social Security Disability Insurance (SSDI) and Supplemental Security Insurance (SSI).[40] And in 1984, the state began full, named reporting of all cases of AIDS.[41] However, state regulations barred hospices and nursing care facilities from admitting people with communicable diseases, which limited the scope of care available to people with AIDS.[42]

Since the state had started compiling lists of people with AIDS, David Jolly began collaborating with the state health department's communicable disease branch to reach people with AIDS.[43] In August, the staff there agreed to send LGHP information to every North Carolinian with AIDS.[44] "We knew that we had to take advantage of [AIDS support organizations'] assistance and their concern," said State Health Director Ron Levine in a later interview, explaining the state's decision to work with the LGHP. "Many individuals, particularly at that stage, were unfamiliar with and afraid of the Health Department or any government-related services, so they were much more comfortable [working with AIDS support organizations]."[45]

The collaboration produced immediate results. According to Dante Noto, the head of LGHP's volunteer services at the time, LGHP soon received "calls from people all over the place: Lumberton, Asheville, it was unbelievable geographic distances."[46] He recalled that "there was probably more of a critical mass in Durham thanks to Duke, but certainly people were coming home from San Francisco and New York back to places like Asheville and Lumberton and other places. And they were in desperate need of support and social services and medical referrals and all the kind of things we did as part of buddy services."[47] By year's end, LGHP volunteers were helping people with AIDS and their families statewide draft wills, find housing, manage household chores, and navigate Social Security.[48] "People forget, . . . it was the *North Carolina* Lesbian and Gay Health Project. It wasn't the Durham health project or the Triangle health project," Noto explained, "it was the only thing."[49]

The upsurge in cases forced the LGHP to develop a more systematic volunteer recruitment system. Initially, recruiting volunteers was easy. "[There were] more people in Durham who looked sick," Adinolfi explained. "People just signed up [to be buddies]. They . . . knew somebody who was sick: had a relative or knew a friend."[50] As AIDS began affecting people outside the local gay community, recruitment began to overwhelm Tony Adinolfi, and by mid-1984 he had recruited Dante Noto to help coordinate AIDS buddies.[51]

Noto and Adinolfi faced two challenges as the AIDS caseload climbed: how could LGHP recruit more "buddies," and how would they train them to cope with the terminal nature of the disease? To address the first, they began advertising for volunteers. "We would run advertisements [in gay newspapers] saying that we were soliciting buddies," explained Noto. "We would go to certain gay social events and let it be known we were looking for buddies. . . . [Then] people would call and offer up their services."[52]

Once someone offered their services, Noto began the training process. Noto conducted an initial interview and then invited the prospect to a training session.[53] Adinolfi and Noto shared this effort, using material gleaned from the Shanti Project and the Gay Men's Health Crisis to help volunteers cope with sorrow and burnout. They also utilized nurses, counselors, other medical professionals, and local hospice staff to train volunteers in their areas of expertise.[54] "We were really close to the hospice people," Adinolfi recalled. "At the time, they wouldn't take AIDS patients . . . but they were good on helping us train on how to care for dying people."[55]

The localized nature of the LGHP, however, made responding to a statewide epidemic difficult. With no paid staff and less than $10,000 in grant support, the LGHP lacked the resources and infrastructure to transform itself into a statewide organization. "We were trying to do the statewide stuff, [but it] was really silly," David Jolly recalled. "Quickly we realized the help we could make was to help other places across the state."[56] Rather than overextending itself, the LGHP opted to assist other gay groups providing AIDS services in their region.

The LGHP played some role in the launch of almost every early AIDS organization in the state. One early group LGHP worked with was in Wilmington.

In the summer of 1983, Gay Resources of Wilmington (GROW), a Wilmington gay social organization, started raising awareness about AIDS. The group's founder, gay activist Leo Teachout, began to warn his community about the disease even before any cases surfaced. In the summer of 1983, Teachout invited LGHP cofounder Carl Wittman to provide his group with an overview of AIDS.[57] The collaboration continued for over a year before Teachout began developing GROW's AIDS services on his own and the LGHP began focusing on other priorities.[58] One of those priorities was helping the AIDS organizing efforts beginning in Charlotte. Cases began surfacing in the summer of 1983, and by the spring of 1984, gay men and their allies launched a relief fund to help mitigate costs incurred by the disease.[59] Strong impetus for this effort came in May of 1984 after a local doctor disclosed the pre-AIDS status of a local nurse to the man's employer, Charlotte Memorial Hospital. When the nurse reported that the hospital had suspended him without pay, Charlotte's gay community rallied around him to provide care and to pursue legal action.[60]

The LGHP helped facilitate these efforts. After the man's partner, Les Kooyman, contacted the LGHP, the LGHP team put his partner in touch with the Lambda Legal Defense and Education Fund.[61] The LGHP team also provided technical assistance to Kooyman so he and his friends could launch what became known as the Metrolina AIDS Project.[62] Over the next eighteen months, gay men and their friends called LGHP for some measure of assistance as they set up AIDS organizations in their local communities. And in this way the LGHP served as an incubator for AIDS organizations in Raleigh, Charlotte, Asheville, Greensboro, Wilmington, and Winston-Salem.[63]

LGHP volunteers also cultivated strong relationships with AIDS clinics. At the UNC School of Medicine, organizing the first AIDS outpatient clinic fell to new junior faculty member Lynn Smiley. While most of Smiley's initial HIV patients came from UNC's hemophilia center, a growing number of AIDS patients came for follow-up after the hospital discharged them. "Then, as word got out that there was this clinic," Smiley recalled, "we got more of these . . . 'well' patients accessing health care at UNC through the clinic rather than from being hospitalized."[64]

White gay men constituted most of these new patients, and as word got out and Smiley established trust, more gay men came to the clinic.[65] "We had more people coming in," Smiley remembered, "so people were getting diagnosed a little bit earlier, before they came in with some full-blown opportunistic infection or something. . . . This was before a lot of the recommendations for how to do counseling. We just sorta had to do it as best we could before the test first came out."[66] As AIDS sparked fear and anxiety among gays and the larger population, many people with AIDS experienced a "terrible isolation": friendships grew awkward and distant, and coworkers stopped their cordial conversations.[67] For Smiley, whose clinic still lacked enough staff to handle the growing number of patients, the arrival of "David Jolly and . . . [the other] volunteers [who] came to the clinic and talked to patients" proved a boon.[68] AIDS clinicians came to rely on the support offered by the LGHP and other AIDS Service Organizations.

The implications of this alliance surfaced over the next year as the HIV antibody test became available. After French researchers discovered HIV in 1983 and the following year American researchers showed that it caused AIDS, the FDA promised to make an antibody test available by the spring of 1985.[69] Various groups responded differently to the news: clinicians expected better management of their patients' disease; epidemiologists anticipated more comprehensive knowledge of the epidemic's scope; and hemophiliacs and blood industry officials hoped it would help protect the nation's blood supply. Gay activists and civil libertarians remained ambivalent, however; they questioned what exposure to the virus meant for someone's "present or future health status"; they feared that housing, custody, insurance, and employment discrimination would ensue if third parties obtained test results and used them against antibody-positive individuals. Thus, in January 1985, even before the FDA released the test, the National Gay Task Force argued that little compensatory benefits accrued to those testing positive, that is, no therapies existed, and recommended that gay men protect their privacy by stopping blood donation, practicing safer sex, and avoiding the antibody test altogether.[70]

For David Jolly and the LGHP volunteers, the National Gay Task Force position posed something of a dilemma. On the one hand, LGHP still relied on breaches in privacy to help patients with AIDS. The agreement with state epidemiologists reinserted a measure of confidentiality into the process, but many referrals would still need to come through word of mouth from friends and medical professionals, particularly for people not fitting the formal definition of an AIDS case. Additionally, David Jolly had at one time wanted North Carolina health officials to keep the contact information of people with "pre-AIDS." ("Unfortunately," Jolly wrote in LGHP's 1984 year-end summary, "North Carolina does not compile a list of people with this condition and we can not reach them as easily as we can people with AIDS").[71] On the other hand, the LGHP shared the "legitimate anxieties" of gay men and lesbians "about the social, economic, and legal consequences of [their] sexual preferences being discovered."[72] While LGHP-related breaches in confidentiality (that is, word-of-mouth referrals) occurred in the context of community solidarity, Jolly feared that indiscriminate use of the antibody test would give health officials, employers, insurance companies, and other vested interests information on thousands of gay men, regardless of their symptoms or infection status, exposing them to untold restrictions and discrimination.[73] Consequently, Jolly and his LGHP colleagues adopted the National Gay Task Force's recommendations. "People should not get the test," Tony Adinolfi explained on behalf of LGHP in March 1985, "because it does not provide clear results and . . . the tests may be available to interested third parties, such as insurance companies or employers."[74]

LGHP's position comported with the stance of other gay groups across the country: since medical professionals and the popular media were conflating AIDS and homosexuality, gay men had a particular interest in protecting their privacy. Gay leaders felt little incentive to sacrifice privacy rights on the altar of public health and viewed coercive health measures as veiled attempts to reassert the "conservative social order."[75] "Having so recently emerged from long, bitter struggles against statutory prohibitions on homosexuality . . . [and] socially sanctioned pattern[s] of discrimination," note HIV chroniclers Ronald Bayer and David Kirp, "it is not surprising that gay political thought was so libertarian in its orientation."[76] Public blame and moralization reinforced this orientation: some conservative observers characterized AIDS as a natural or supernatural judgment; others blamed the epidemic on "self-indulgent" homosexuals and drug users.[77] Concerns over infection by "routine household contact" turned this public chastisement into panic, recrimination, and discrimination.[78] In this tense environment, gay leaders forecasted "horror scenario[s]" in which "government officials" would quarantine all the gay men exposed to the virus.[79] Gays' fears were not unfounded, as cases of discrimination against gays and people with AIDS rose rapidly between 1983 and 1985: several North Carolina men lost their jobs, housing, health insurance, and parental rights because they had AIDS or they were presumed to have AIDS.[80] It was within this context that David Jolly and other LGHP staff forged their position on testing and privacy.

It was also in this context that North Carolina's public health officials forged their AIDS response. Some, in North Carolina as elsewhere, adhered to traditional public health strategies that targeted, tested, and traced those at risk in order to contain the virus within the smallest population possible; for them, HIV infection was like any other communicable disease.[81] A more influential group of public health leaders argued that coercive measures would drive those at risk "underground" and championed instead an "exceptionalist," position that controlled HIV infection through voluntary, anonymous, patient-initiated testing; community-based prevention; and other noncoercive interventions.[82]

This "exceptionalism" faction gained the upper hand in North Carolina largely due to the influence of the state's communicable disease director, Dr. Rebecca Meriwether.[83] Reared in Tennessee and trained in Georgia, Meriwether came to work for the North Carolina Health Department in the early 1980s. Her coworkers there found her "really smart and really progressive in terms of public health" and even, according to gay activists, "very pro-gay."[84] Consequently, Meriwether favored creating alternative sites for people to undergo anonymous antibody tests, believing that—in the absence of robust antidiscrimination provisions—traditional health measures would thwart gay men's privacy rights and drive them from mainstream medical care.[85] The most effective way to ensure that gay men supported prevention efforts, Meriwether believed, was to cooperate with them rather than impose "solutions" on them.[86]

Jolly and his LGHP colleagues confirmed Meriwether's suspicions. In the spring of 1985, as the FDA prepared to release the tests, Meriwether met with Jolly and Adinolfi to gauge their support of an anonymous testing option.[87] Jolly and Adinolfi explained their recommendation to avoid the test, but they expressed willingness to collaborate on anonymous testing, pre- and post-test counseling, and ways that the "LGHP and [the STD-]control people could cooperate" in the future.[88]

With members of the gay community cautiously on board, Meriwether sold the plan to her boss, state health director Ronald Levine, who in turn convinced the North Carolina Health Commission to adopt the strategy. "The [commission] relied heavily on me," Levine remembered, "[and] I relied heavily on a superb staff." The step was not without controversy, however. "No one ever heard of such a thing," Levine recalled. "'Anonymous testing? What kind of business is that?' . . . I really got leaned on hard. . . . [Many health workers wondered], 'Why can't we treat AIDS like any other communicable disease?' . . . [and] attacked us very strongly. . . . Some of them were my friends, and they were very, very upset and angry."[89] The emphasis on patient-initiated testing ran against so much of what these physicians considered to be the best way to address an epidemic. Despite the opposition, however, Levine trusted Meriwether on anonymous testing: "We felt it was important; the staff said it was critical. We had a budding crisis on our hands.

. . . [There were] questions surrounding the adequacy of confidentiality, . . . fear of going to a 'government' agency, . . . fears of discrimination, many of which were well-founded. . . . [So] we came up with this anonymous testing. . . . [and] the commission was great . . . they followed our lead; we argued strongly for anonymous testing, [and] I think it was highly successful."[90]

In short order, North Carolina launched one of the most widespread testing plans in the country. "[Meriwether] felt like [North Carolina] needed to normalize [AIDS] and that every health department in the state should be dealing with it whether they like it or not," David Jolly explained. "So she was instrumental in getting HIV testing done in every health department in the state."[91] Using federal and state funds, the state opened its first alternate testing facility in May (North Carolina's Red Cross centers received their tests in mid-March after high-risk areas like New York and San Francisco received their test kits first), and by year's end, the Health Department had opened testing facilities—with free anonymous testing with pre- and post-test counseling—in ninety-four counties.[92] Anonymous testing sites were more accessible in North Carolina than in New York City.[93]

North Carolina's blood industry supported these efforts. Industry officials watched as media reports in early 1985 stoked public fears about blood safety, driving down blood donations. Industry officials also worried about high-risk donors who received a false negative on their test and inadvertently introduced infected blood into the blood supply. Alternative testing sites were therefore in the industry's interest, and groups like the Red Cross actively supported them in North Carolina.[94] "It would be a very serious problem to have high-risk individuals donating blood simply to get the results of this screening test, which may fail in some cases," Red Cross regional director Dr. Jerry Squires explained to reporters. "These individuals should avail themselves of medical follow-up. . . . They should understand we are not providing them with any kind of a terminal prognosis. This test doesn't do that."[95] "This is not a test for AIDS," added Dr. J. N. MacCormack, chief of the Health Department's infectious disease branch. "We frankly don't know what it means, except that the antibodies to the virus are present and that blood from that individual shouldn't be used. One thing we ought to be thinking here is the potential mental health problem that could [develop] from this screening test."[96] "We don't want to see someone donating blood to get this test and then killing himself based on the results," concluded LGHP's Tony Adinolfi.[97] As the state's alternate testing program rolled out, AIDS activists, blood industry leaders, and public health officials spoke with one voice: protect people's privacy and mental health as well as the blood supply. An alliance around AIDS exceptionalism had been forged in North Carolina.

IT IS IMPORTANT AT THIS STAGE to reflect on the health policy implications of the actions taken by Health Department officials. Many health policy researchers believe health policy research should concentrate on the way governments allocate scarce resources for health, while others emphasize the structure and delivery of health services or the determinants of health in health outcomes. I embrace health policy scholar Gill Walt's contention that health policy "is synonymous with politics," that it "deals explicitly with who influences policy making, how they exercise that influence, under what conditions."[98] The AIDS mobilization discussed above is important because it highlights the way "courses of action . . . affect the set of institutions, organizations, services, and funding arrangements of the health system."[99] In this case, policy choices outside North Carolina (such as the support of AIDS exceptionalism by activists and health officials in places like San Francisco and New York) combined with policy allegiances inside the state to generate AIDS policies of a particular sort, and this had particular consequences for the shape of AIDS in North Carolina.

North Carolina's anonymous testing scheme, which prioritized blood-supply protection and awareness-raising rather than surveillance and prevention, was one such policy. Health officials adopted an approach to antibody testing that protected the blood supply but also created a safe space—voluntary, anonymous testing—for awareness to occur. The trade-offs of this system were that it inhibited accurate surveillance of the epidemic (it had a selection bias: only those aware of their risk and the available resources availed themselves of the test), and it made prevention more difficult (anonymous testing made contact tracing challenging, and the data it produced reflected where the epidemic had already been, not where it was going next). Importantly, this scheme also was based on certain assumptions about the population's risk for HIV infection: based on the available state and U.S. data, public health officials assumed gay men were at greatest risk for infection. They also assumed that most of these men had or could obtain adequate health care, and that they would access this health care system (i.e., not go underground) if health practitioners avoided overly coercive measures. While North Carolina public health officials lacked evidence indicating these things were true or would actually occur, they heeded the LGHP team's warnings that high-risk gay men would, in fact, drop out of the system if coercive measures were in place.

Just as the shape of testing policy prioritized the concerns of white gay men, so too did the developing AIDS care and support structure. While LGHP volunteers knew AIDS affected others, white gay men accounted for all the cases they saw in 1983 and 1984. Consequently, most of the early volunteers with the LGHP were white gay men and their friends and allies. Most of the volunteer recruiting took place in gay bars, among gay-affirming groups, through gay social networks, and in the gay media. Volunteers, therefore, came largely out of a relationship-based (rather than kinship-, religion-, or class-based) social network. Moreover, since state health officials had started relying on the LGHP for advice on AIDS, and since the LGHP largely saw AIDS as a threat to white gay men, the state focused its attention in this direction. Indeed, in 1986 the state hired David Jolly to run its AIDS effort.

State statistics seemed to support this attention, since reporting delays about AIDS in minority communities inflated the proportionate severity of the epidemic among white gays in the state.[100] AIDS did not become officially reportable in North Carolina until 1984, so physicians reported fewer than 60 percent of all the AIDS cases diagnosed in North Carolina prior to that, and none of those reported cases involved African Americans. Thus, in these early years, the AIDS epidemic appeared largely white to the North Carolina Health Department and the CDC. Even after the Health Commission required AIDS reporting, it took several years before the extent of AIDS among African Americans became apparent. Health officials, media outlets, and service organizations had little way to know that AIDS was already disproportionately affecting African Americans. Consequently, the state's early program largely reflected the national discourse around AIDS, which focused on the problem of AIDS in white gay communities and relied on strategies tested or vetted by white AIDS activists.[101] Jolly's hiring reinforced this.

From 1983, however, the disease had taken root in other communities in North Carolina.[102] African Americans, for example, actually bore a disproportionate share of the disease. Though blacks constituted only 22 percent of the population, 42 percent of the cases diagnosed in 1983 occurred among African Americans.[103] Moreover, while sex between men constituted the most common means of exposure, a growing number of cases were occurring among women and among injection drug users.[104]

The most rapidly expanding risk group in these years was African Americans. By 1985, African Americans in North Carolina accounted for more new AIDS cases than whites (fig. 2.1). And in contrast to white communities, where AIDS largely occurred among men who have sex with men (MSM), drug use posed as great a transmission risk as MSM for African Americans

FIGURE 2.1. North Carolina HIV/AIDS Cases by Race, 1983–1985

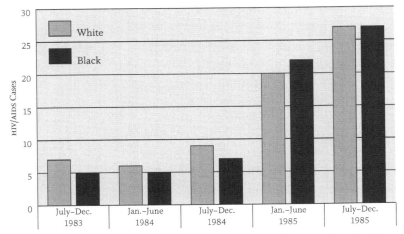

Source: U.S. Department of Health and Human Services, Centers for Disease Control and Prevention, National Center for HIV, STD and TB Prevention, AIDS Public Information Data Set, U.S. Surveillance Data for 1981–2002, CDC WONDER Downloadable Database, software version 2.7.1, December 2005.

(tables 2.1 and 2.2). Moreover, blacks who acquired HIV tended to be poorer and have more limited access to medical care than white people with AIDS. White gays rapidly spread rudimentary AIDS awareness throughout their social networks, giving gay men a basic checklist of AIDS symptomatology. So by the mid-1980s, concerned white gay men began availing themselves of the outpatient AIDS clinics that opened at places like North Carolina Memorial Hospital and Duke Medical Center.[105] African Americans—whether MSM, drug users, or other high-risk individuals—lacked a grassroots push for this type of self-surveillance. This meant that physicians in North Carolina tended to diagnose AIDS in African American patients much later in the disease's progression than white patients, often only after a severe AIDS-related health emergency put them in the hospital.

From early in the epidemic, African Americans in North Carolina experienced a more diverse and numerically more severe epidemic than whites, yet this did not translate into policymaking power. The leadership of the LGHP remained white, as did the top circles of management in North Carolina's Health Department and blood industry. Black gay groups had not come forward to champion their needs, if they were even aware of them, and few black physicians recognized the threat that AIDS posed to members in black communities. Thus the AIDS alliance that mobilized in these early years lacked

TABLE 2.1. White AIDS Cases by Transmission Factor in Major
North Carolina Cities, 1981–1989

	MSM	MSM Intravenous Drug User	Intravenous Drug User	Hetero-sexual	Blood Recipient	Hemo-philiac	Un-disclosed
1981							
1982	2						
1983	6	1					1
1984	11	1					
1985	19	1		1	2	1	
1986	39	1	4	2	4	3	2
1987	78	3	9	1	6	5	
1988	76		11	2	5	3	5
1989	106	8	15	1	1	4	9

Source: U.S. Department of Health and Human Services, Centers for Disease Control and Prevention, National Center for HIV, STD and TB Prevention, AIDS Public Information Data Set, U.S. Surveillance Data for 1981–2002, CDC WONDER Online Database, December 2005, http://wonder.cdc.gov/aids-v2002.html.

TABLE 2.2. Black AIDS Cases by Transmission Factor in Major
North Carolina Cities, 1981–1989

	MSM	MSM Intravenous Drug User	Intravenous Drug User	Hetero-sexual	Blood Recipient	Hemo-philiac	Un-disclosed
1981			1				
1982							
1983			2				
1984	5	3			1		
1985	12	7	2	1	1	2	
1986	11	11	4		1		2
1987	30	30	6	6	1	1	3
1988	45	44	5	14	3	1	2
1989	51	69	18	20	2	1	7

Source: See Table 2.1.

substantive representation from African Americans, and the policy responses that grew out of this alliance largely reflected the white, middle-class, gay concerns from which they came. What remained to be seen, however, was the extent to which policies crafted out of this cultural context best served the growing number of African Americans affected by the AIDS epidemic. North Carolina's testing and surveillance program was commendable, but it relied on community awareness and access to mainstream health care. Such a strategy proved ineffectual for people who already existed at the margins of the health care system and were unaware of their own risk. From the start of the epidemic, then, poverty, drug use, AIDS awareness, and poor health care access all worked together to influence the contours of the epidemic in African American communities.

CHAPTER 3

WE AIN'T GOING TO TELL NOBODY
AIDS Organizations and the Challenge of Diversity

Louise Alston and her family shuffled into the elevator on an evening in late November 1986. No one spoke. Each family member weighed the tragic news they had just learned: Harold Burton, Louise's brother, had AIDS. That morning, Harold had gone to the hospital to have his teeth removed, and by evening he was telling his parents and five siblings that he had a terminal disease. Louise knew something about HIV because of her work as a phlebotomist, so she tried calming her family's fears about AIDS; but everyone still felt panicked. Now, standing together in stunned silence, each seemed to be pondering what to do next. Finally, from the back of the elevator, Louise's father spoke. "We ain't going to tell nobody what he got," Mr. Burton said. "We goin' to say that he's sick from his diabetes."[1] Silence again filled the elevator. But the solution unsettled Louise. She placed her hand gently on his shoulder. "Daddy," she said in her deeply calming voice, "That's not the answer. That's not the answer."[2]

BY 1986, THE SPREAD of HIV/AIDS forced hundreds of families across North Carolina to determine their response to the disease. Black families like the Burtons often found themselves alone and confused about what to do or say. At that point in time, few black organizations were equipped to deal with AIDS, and the social stigmas associated with the disease pressured many families to suffer in silence. For a host of reasons, white gay organizations would not prove to be the most effective platforms for addressing AIDS in minority communities. Moreover, their constant battles with social conservatives at both the state and local levels often narrowed the scope of their policy priorities to ones that privileged self-preservation. While this made sense for them, it would have important implications for the shape of HIV policies in the state. Between 1986 and 1989, however, the social landscape of the disease changed as a growing number of individuals and families began dealing with AIDS, and a growing number of mainstream community groups—

including minority and substance abuse programs—joined gay organizations in the fight against AIDS in the state. This chapter explores the development of those efforts, the effect they had, and the challenges faced by the groups raising AIDS awareness in African American communities.

AIDS organizations had not ignored African Americans, but their outreach efforts had thus far proven ineffective. In 1986, for example, the Lesbian and Gay Health Project (LGHP) had recruited several minorities to help diversify its membership and better reach minority communities. Between 1986 and 1987, LGHP recruited three minority men to work with the group, one Asian (Lester Lee) and two African Americans (Gary Lipscomb and Godfrey Herndon).[3] The LGHP's main AIDS educator, Scott Hustead, also emphasized minority outreach.[4] These efforts notwithstanding, the LGHP had little success reaching black gays. Dating circles largely remained segregated in Durham, and many gay blacks thought white gays cared little for blacks or their freedom struggle.[5] Moreover, many black gays, who enjoyed little support from the larger black community, chose to hide their sexual orientation, preserving a hypermasculine public image while participating in covert male-only sexual networks.[6] This clandestine and ambiguous sexual identity kept many blacks outside mainstream gay culture and made them hard to reach by the state's largely white AIDS groups. Many black gay social networks were even closed to Garry Lipscomb, one of the black volunteers working with the LGHP, because of his connections to a white gay organization.[7] As early as 1986 and 1987, it became clear that effective prevention among black men who have sex with men (MSM) would prove exceedingly difficult for "white" AIDS organizations.

IN THE MID-1980S black groups in North Carolina had yet to embrace the threat of AIDS or mobilize private capital, public resources, and popular media to tackle the problem. African Americans who became aware of AIDS did so up close—as families dealing with a catastrophic illness. And like many catastrophic illnesses, AIDS caught many families off guard. This was true for Harold Burton's family: they knew no one with AIDS, they had little inkling of its prevalence among African Americans, and they were unaware that Burton's life and lifestyle—his drug use, poor health, poverty, needle sharing, and frequent travel to coastal cities—put him at risk for this disease that affected white gays.

Burton himself clearly was unaware of his risk as well. In 1986, his health had declined, but he attributed it to his diabetes and drug use. Since North Carolina utilized an opt-in voluntary testing scheme, Burton never asked for an HIV test. It was not until one of his scheduled medical visits that year that an astute resident who was aware of Burton's history of drug use suggested he had HIV. Skirting consent requirements, Burton's physician used a surrogate test to discover Burton's CD4 count to be well below 200. He immediately diagnosed Burton with "full blown AIDS" and, without counseling Burton about the meaning of the test or the syndrome itself, arranged for Burton's admission to the community hospital. It was only after his sister, Louise Alston, arrived at the hospital to begin caring for him that he learned the truth.[8] As was the case with many other African Americans in his situation, Burton did not know about the LGHP, nor were there any black organizations to which he or his family could really turn for help. His experience highlights the extent to which few community resources had been devoted to raising awareness about and providing care for AIDS in African American communities.

There were, of course, plenty of places where the interests of people with AIDS overlapped, regardless of their race or the means by which they acquired the infection. Providing care for people who were diagnosed with the disease proved to be one of the most pressing areas of concern. AIDS terrified or repulsed many medical professionals, particularly in the early years when uncertainty existed about transmission routes and outrageous fears and stigma prevailed. Sometimes physicians and hospitals refused to see people with AIDS altogether: in 1985, one rural hospital in North Carolina refused to treat a patient with AIDS and sent him via ambulance to North Carolina Memorial Hospital wrapped in a body bag with a straw as an airvent.[9] Obviously this was an extreme response, but many doctors in the state routinely declined to treat those with AIDS and directed them to other physicians.[10] The practice became so common that in 1987 the North Carolina Medical Society demanded that all its members "render quality health care to patients with AIDS."[11]

Other medical professionals responded similarly. "We would go to regional meetings," David Jolly later recalled, "and health department people would come in. . . . Some of them were absolutely wonderful—but there were a bunch of them that . . . did not want to touch this issue with a stick and . . . if they had any choice they would not have been there. Gay people were just 'sick' and . . . there was racial prejudice. They would talk about their clients with disdain. . . . There was terrific disdain."[12] Funeral home directors proved a particular problem. One woman became so distraught at a funeral home's refusal to take her husband's body that she pleaded with her husband's clinician for help. Lynn Smiley, director of UNC's AIDS clinic, convinced the funeral director to take the man's body. "He was just operating out of ignorance," Smiley later recalled, "because the universal precautions thing hadn't rolled into his profession yet."[13] For many families in the mid-1980s, the gap between daily practice and professional responsibility seemed particularly cruel.

Improving the care that patients with AIDS received became an issue on several fronts. As mentioned in the previous chapter, gay-originated AIDS organizations like the LGHP filled the void at the local level in many communities. In communities lacking an organized gay presence—like Cumberland County, which had accumulated the third highest number of HIV/AIDS cases in the state by 1986—groups of health care workers came together with concerned citizens to form AIDS task forces to ensure that people with AIDS received adequate care in the county. Efforts also occurred at the state level. From his position in the state's public health service, David Jolly pushed for more compassionate responses. Additionally, a loosely coordinated group of gay AIDS workers launched a political action committee (dubbed the AIDS Services Coalition [ASC]) to encourage benevolent AIDS policies in the state. The group, led by Metrolina AIDS Project (MAP) director Les Kooyman, represented AIDS workers on the state's AIDS task force and lobbied legislators at the state capitol.[14] A variety of medical professionals joined this effort. Across the state then, in 1986 and 1987, several communities began working to humanize the response to people with AIDS.

Conceivably, this emphasis on improving care could have brought African American groups into the AIDS effort, but this never happened. Having agreed to care for her ailing brother, Alston smacked up against the shoddy care that many hospitals were providing patients with AIDS. At Durham Regional Hospital, where Burton stayed the first weeks after his diagnosis, hospital staff donned full infection-control garb upon entering his room. Some staff refused to enter his room altogether, and Alston frequently found Harold's meals outside his door and his trash can overflowing when she came to visit. One afternoon, after learning that Burton had missed two meals and had yet to receive his insulin shots, Alston loudly confronted hospital administrators. "This is unacceptable," she yelled, banging repeatedly on the counter at the nurse's station. "The boy is a drug user, if you give him his needle he can . . . take his insulin. And why is his food put on the floor here? . . . He is so weak now he cannot get up. I will not have this. I will have your heads for it. You are in the profession! You take the good with the bad!"[15] Burton received better care thereafter, but Alston never lost that bitter memory. What was important, from Alston's perspective, was that she had to fight for Burton's care on her own.

Part of the reason that AIDS organizations struggled to diversify in 1987 was that AIDS became profoundly politicized, at both state and national levels. Many white gay organizations in North Carolina found themselves fighting a rear-guard action against social conservatives over the content of AIDS education curriculums, the nature and content of AIDS prevention strategies, and the identity of AIDS organizations. Prior to 1987, social conservatives in North Carolina had largely ignored HIV/AIDS as a political issue, most likely because they did not consider the issue to have much relevance for the state. Concerns over sex education changed their perspective, however. In late 1986, many school boards began proposing that AIDS-specific information be included in the state's sex-education curriculum.[16] In response, David Jolly announced in early 1987 that his office would draft a model AIDS curriculum for school boards to adopt.[17] The prospect of a state-sponsored AIDS curriculum concerned some conservatives, and so in mid-April, state representative Coy Privette and some conservative colleagues floated a bill in the state legislature that promised to maintain control over the content by requiring the state curriculum to stress abstinence, discuss sex only within the context of marriage, and deemphasize condoms and other prevention methods.[18] The bill sparked lengthy debate during the following months: many Republicans supported the measure, while several Democrats called for a more "realistic" and comprehensive curriculum that provided kids with complete prophylactic information. Ultimately, legislators landed in the middle, leaving the specific content to the state school board but requiring that the final product stress "parental involvement," "abstinence education," and "other accurate and appropriate information to prevent the spread of the disease." The school board complied, neutralizing Jolly's original "gay-positive, sex positive" curriculum so that it emphasized abstinence and life-long monogamy while still including prophylaxis education. The compromise and ensuing curriculum left neither conservatives nor liberals truly satisfied (Privette's camp wanted the curriculum to go further in a conservative direction while state liberals felt it already went too far). By the end of 1987, North Carolina had become one of only sixteen states with mandatory public AIDS instruction.[19]

Privette and his colleagues were also concerned about the state's surveillance and control measures. North Carolina's Health Department had adopted a voluntary, anonymous testing regime across the state in 1985. By 1987, the department had hired two specialists to track down unreported AIDS cases in the state, and it also began training health professionals on AIDS care, surveillance, and control procedures.[20] Tapping into the sentiments of many health practitioners, Privette and his colleagues called for a return to more traditional control and containment strategies. AIDS should be treated like any other communicable disease, they maintained, and not as an excuse to extend gay rights at the expense of public health. Privette and his allies recommended the use of quarantine powers and the mandatory testing of prisoners, sex workers, food handlers, and engaged couples.[21] Opponents acknowledged that such coercive measures might in some "exceptionally rare case" protect the public good, but they argued that in most cases such programs would "harm the public health by driving those most at risk of infection into defensive postures."[22] These exceptionalist, or noncoercive, arguments convinced most state lawmakers, and, save for granting the health director emergency quarantine powers, none of Privette's proposed measures passed.[23]

Undeterred, Privette and his conservative allies took their campaign to the state's newly formed AIDS task force. The governor had established the task force to provide guidance on the most pressing concerns related to AIDS and to make recommendations on the best ways to invest AIDS money that the Centers for Disease Control and Prevention (CDC) began offering to states. To obtain these federal funds, states had to show the CDC that they had implemented partner-notification plans.[24] North Carolina had opted not to implement such plans when it established its testing program in 1985, but by 1987, significant money was now available from the government and at least one AIDS drug, AZT, showed tremendous therapeutic potential, so a growing chorus of voices began calling for contact tracing. Consequently, the AIDS task force began working with the Health Department to put contact tracing in place.[25]

It was at this point that Privette and his colleagues sought to influence policy. They began pressuring task force members to implement mandatory contact tracing and to levy fines against or quarantine noncompliant patients. For some task force members, such policy options were not totally unwelcome. "[Contact tracing is] very expensive and controversial," acknowledged task force member Dr. Cheryl McCartney, "but because of recent findings that infectivity varies at various times, that makes it even more important to notify contacts."[26]

In response, health workers, AIDS activists, and civil libertarians mobilized against the proposal. David Jolly and his allies within the Health Department worked to defeat the proposals. "Contact tracing would not enhance our current efforts to control AIDS," Jolly told legislators in February 1987. "[It] would direct important resources away from the education of high-risk groups and the general public."[27] The North Carolina Civil Liberties Union highlighted the deficiencies in the plan and called for greater investment in prevention.[28] AIDS activists like Les Kooyman, who served both as the head of Metrolina AIDS Project and as a member of the AIDS task force, argued in public forums that mandatory contact tracing would "drive [the disease] underground" and that punishing "non-compliant" patients would end gay men's cooperation with the state.[29] Such a punitive proposal, argued Larry Gostin of the American Society for Law and Medicine, departed from "everything we know about public health and contact tracing."[30] David Jones, a retired pharmaceutical executive who was lobbying on behalf of the Lesbian and Gay Health Project, went door to door at the state capitol to convince lawmakers to oppose the measures and demanded that the governor add a person with AIDS to the task force.[31]

With such strong opposition, the task force backed away from the mandatory contact tracing proposal and accepted a plan offered by Rebecca Meriwether and David Jolly for voluntary, anonymous contact tracing.[32] The "opt-in" tracing mechanism allowed people to report their contacts directly to a health professional or anonymously by mail. Moreover, physicians were not required to tell a patient's spouse if the patient tested positive; they could leave it up to a patient if they felt the patient would comply, but could also have the public health department inform the spouse if they felt the patient would not comply.[33] Additionally, a person with AIDS was appointed to the task force to "bring a real-world perspective on what [people with AIDS] face."[34] AIDS activists had prevented Privette and his colleagues from implementing mandatory reporting and tracing in North Carolina.

The debates about AIDS and identity also played out at the local level. In 1985, gay men in Charlotte had founded the Metrolina AIDS Project (MAP). Though it was an AIDS organization ostensibly serving all people with AIDS and not just gay men, it largely retained a gay cultural identity and mainly serviced gay men with the disease. With AIDS on the rise in Mecklenburg County (70 percent of Charlotte's fifty-five AIDS cases surfaced between 1986 and 1987), local officials routinely relied on the group to address the city's burgeoning epidemic.[35] This growing prominence encouraged MAP to seek funds from the city in its efforts against AIDS. "We're asking to become . . . part of the established community network of services in Mecklenburg County," MAP director Les Kooyman explained in his petition for county funds in the summer of 1987.[36] In June 1987, commissioners agreed, giving Metrolina $33,613 toward their budget and bringing the group into Charlotte's social service network.

Controversy quickly enveloped the group, however. From its founding,

MAP had committed itself to upholding a gay-positive and sex-positive message focused on harm reduction. Like countless groups across the country, MAP frequently handed out "safer-sex cards" at gay bars that listed risk levels of sexual behaviors on one side and contact information on the other. In December 1987, a local pastor and leader of an antipornography group, the Reverend Joseph Chambers, learned about the cards and complained to the county commissioners. After officials orchestrated a meeting, MAP agreed to stop distributing the cards and to submit all future handout materials for county approval. Dissatisfied with this compromise, Chambers took his complaints public, labeling MAP "a homosexual club" and demanding that commissioners defund the project and transfer all AIDS funds to the Health Department.[37] The commission ignored his complaint and merely reiterated the December agreement that required MAP to clear its materials with the Health Department. "This is the only game in town," one commissioner explained. "This is all we've got and we need to support it."[38] Seventy-five letters of support came from the community defending MAP, and several physicians voiced their support.[39] Those opposed to the group—including some commissioners and the county health director—lost out to the majority of commissioners who found the cards appropriate for AIDS prevention among gay men. "Not only do I think we should fund [MAP]," explained one supportive commissioner; "I think we ought to be thinking about more money for it."[40] While Chambers hoped to marginalize MAP, in fact the Chambers controversy helped establish MAP as part of the Charlotte's mainstream service structure.

This kind of controversy only reinforced the fears gay men had about conservative intentions to roll back gay rights under the pretext of public health. With legislators calling for mandatory tracing and threatening to implement fines or imprisonment for noncompliance, gay men put no confidence in North Carolina's confidentiality provisions and had little interest entrusting their names or the names of their sexual partners to the Health Department. Consequently, beginning in 1987, gay activists formally organized their lobbying efforts against what they believed to be punitive and obstructionist AIDS policies. David Jones, the retired pharmaceutical executive who had led the lobbying effort at the state capitol, left his volunteer position with the Lesbian and Gay Health Project to lobby formally for the AIDS Services Coalition.[41]

The ASC's priorities were to protect the privacy of people with HIV, create a continuum of care for people with AIDS, and get people with AIDS and AIDS activists onto decision-making committees. The battle over the acceptability of MAP in Charlotte signified the toxic environment in which the problem of AIDS existed: people routinely conflated homosexuality and AIDS and stigmatized both. Consequently, over the next year, Jones and his allies began working on an anti-discrimination bill. They also pushed several informed-consent measures and fought endlessly to raise state AIDS appropriations.

Over the next several years, the main AIDS-related policy debates in the state centered on the issues of privacy, surveillance, and disease control. Even as the epidemic itself diversified, the public discourse and policy responses became polarized. Such a politicized atmosphere made working toward a more polyphonic response—one that might effectively draw minorities and others into the AIDS effort—more difficult to achieve.

While white gays held the most influence over AIDS policy-setting in the state, the growing diversity of the epidemic expanded the pool of interested parties beyond gay communities. Several other groups emerged during this period to address the growing needs of those affected by AIDS. In 1987, for example, the Episcopal Diocese, the Unitarian-Universalists, and Triangle Hospice began working with LGHP volunteers to find housing in Durham for people with AIDS.[42] AIDS frequently left people without adequate housing for a variety of reasons: the disease might leave someone unable to afford their rent; fear of the disease might get someone barred from their prior housing; or the severity of the disease might necessitate a level of nursing care unavailable to them in other contexts. In the second half of the 1980s, the state had yet to make provisions for such people. The problem grew more intense as people from across the nation came to North Carolina's hospitals for treatment. Visitors frequently could not afford housing or find temporary places to live, and some "slept in the phone booths they used to call AIDS associations for help."[43] On May 1, 1988, the newly dubbed AIDS Community Residence Association (ACRA) purchased a five-bedroom house in the Durham area to retrofit for AIDS patients.[44] ACRA hoped to care for six patients at a time in the house while providing emergency rent and utility funds for others with HIV/AIDS.[45]

Other organizations stepped up their efforts as well. Church-related groups had cared for people with AIDS from the beginning of the epidemic, and several religious groups provided the backbone of care for buddy programs and housing efforts. Clergy sat on AIDS task forces across the state, parishioners frequently volunteered with AIDS groups, and several churches launched AIDS ministries and clergy training seminars.[46] People in rural counties likewise began addressing the problem. In 1987, for example, the number of people with AIDS in rural Burke County rose. With no gay groups active in the area, the staff at the Burke County Health Department and Grace Hospital joined local clergy, teachers, and concerned citizens to form the Burke County AIDS Task Force. By 1988, the task force, renamed the AIDS Leadership Foothills-Area Alliance (ALFA), secured a $1,000 grant from the United Way to provide AIDS services to people in several adjoining counties.[47] Similar projects were launched in Asheville (Western North Carolina [WNC] AIDS Project) and Greenville (Eastern Regional AIDS Support and Education [ERASE]).[48]

It was these other organizations that ultimately brought black communities and health workers into the effort against AIDS. In mid-1986, black staff members at the Durham branch of the Red Cross recognized that few AIDS outreach programs specifically targeted African Americans. Since 1986 surveillance numbers were beginning to show the disproportionate impact of HIV on blacks, these workers sensed the threat that AIDS posed to members of their community.[49] To begin sounding the alarm about AIDS, the Red Cross staff partnered with a prominent black physician in the area, Dr. Elaine Hart-Brothers, to educate local black medical professionals about AIDS.[50] These seminars prompted Dr. Howard Fitts, head of health education at North Carolina Central University and chair of the health committee for the politically powerful Durham Committee for the Affairs of Black People (DCABP), to launch an AIDS-awareness campaign in the Triangle's black communities. In February 1987, Fitts and Deborah Giles, a substance abuse nurse who sat on the committee, held a community forum to raise awareness about AIDS in African American communities.[51]

Over the next year, Fitts and the DCABP increased their efforts to warn local black communities about AIDS.[52] They found few resources that were culturally competent for African Americans: most AIDS prevention strategies had been developed by and for white gay men, and few research studies had explored how African American communities balanced their racial, social, and sexual identities in light of AIDS.[53] Fitts found that those most affected by AIDS in black communities— gays and injection drug users— lacked the infrastructure to organize. Fitts also recognized that white groups had failed to reach at-risk blacks and that African American organizations had been reluctant to pick up the slack.[54] Public health workers had tried to draft culturally appropriate AIDS material—David Jolly had adapted an AIDS pamphlet for general use from a black gay and lesbian organization in Baltimore, for example—but most often they simply transplanted programs that worked among white gays into minority communities.[55] Fitts felt that these programs translated poorly, however, and most of the research evaluating these programs led to the same conclusion.[56] Fitts and his team set out to find AIDS outreach programs in other parts of the country that had effectively reached minorities, and they began planning an AIDS clearinghouse to provide information and resources on AIDS interventions that worked in black communities.

Launching a black AIDS organization was no easy task, however. Several fledgling efforts had emerged across the state in 1987. In Wilmington, a black public health worker launched the AIDS Awareness in the Black Community Project (AABC); in Charlotte, an interracial program began addressing minority AIDS in the city; in High Point, a black church started an AIDS ministry for local families; and in Raleigh, Shaw University held an AIDS conference for black churches dealing with AIDS.[57] But these were small-scale efforts, and it was a struggle to keep them going.

Meanwhile, oblivious to Dr. Fitts's effort in Durham, Louise Alston began a campaign with her recuperating brother to raise AIDS awareness among Burton's previous sexual and needle-sharing partners. Beginning in 1987, Alston and Burton "started going to the communities he hung out with using drugs . . . to talk to the people about not sharing the needles like [Burton] did."[58] Since Burton continued using drugs even after his diagnosis, finding many of his previous contacts proved easy. Their message about not sharing needles found little reception, however. "[Burton] didn't look sick," Alston recalled. "He was still walking around, he was still being funny, he was still using drugs, and they thought, 'So, ain't nothing wrong with you. Nothing wrong with you.'"[59] When Burton did grow ill, most of his peers ascribed it to his diabetes.[60] Burton and Alston made little headway encouraging users to get tested or to follow up on potential symptoms. By the time most users became aware of HIV/AIDS, it was far too late.[61] In the meantime, Alston and Burton were never able to translate their efforts into a more sustainable program. Without community buy-in and support, most of these efforts lacked the resources to have much impact.

BUILDING A SUSTAINABLE MINORITY AIDS program became more possible by the end of 1987, however, after state health officials displayed a growing awareness of racial health disparities in general and the disproportionate AIDS burden in particular. Health workers in the state "started talking about racial disparities in the late 80s," David Jolly recalled. "There was an office of minority health that was set up that reported to Ron Levine . . . [and] there was increasing awareness that [the AIDS-control program] needed to do more in the African American community."[62] In 1987, the state health department applied for and obtained $170,000 in grants from the CDC. After some political machinations, by the summer of 1988, the Department of Health had had hired three black health workers—to improve contact with minority communities—and released the rest of the money to host several AIDS conferences and fund eleven AIDS programs across the state.[63] Five of these outreach programs specifically targeted black communities, and three others addressed injection drug use—a problem particularly prevalent among African Americans.[64]

Howard Fitts and the Durham Committee received some of these state funds. Fitts and his team contended that African Americans had largely disregarded AIDS warnings because "aspects of AIDS education . . . may be peculiar to black populations."[65] In his application for funds, Fitts proposed that the Durham Committee would establish an AIDS Clearinghouse to provide accurate AIDS information to minority communities in ten counties surrounding Durham.[66] It would serve as the foundation for an AIDS resource network, with AIDS educators reaching out to high-risk groups.[67] Fitts hired a full-time public health educator and a part-time administrative assistant to launch the program in the summer of 1988. Durham and the surrounding counties finally had an AIDS Service Organization devoted specifically to the needs of African Americans. It was one of five programs in the state specifically targeting African American communities.[68]

Another program receiving funds was the Durham County Health Department's harm reduction program for injection drug users called Project Straighttalk. Because of the controversy surrounding the disease and its seemingly tangential connection to drug addiction, substance abuse professionals in North Carolina had largely avoided the AIDS issue in the early 1980s. "There was too much stigma attached," recalled David Jolly. "What they said to us was 'this is a public health issue, not a substance abuse issue.' . . . They felt like their plate was already full just dealing with flat-out, old-fashioned substance abuse that they didn't have enough time, energy, or resources. . . . It was just a matter of time before they had to deal with it. But we struggled mightily [in] '86, '87, '88 to work with them, to get them to pay any attention at all."[69] By 1988, addiction specialists had come around, however. "It was inevitable," Jolly recalled, "it was just a matter of time before they had to deal with it."[70] The connection between substance abuse and HIV/AIDS could not be ignored: the number of users with AIDS tripled between 1986 and 1988, and injection drug users had come to account for one-quarter of AIDS cases in the state.[71] To respond to Durham's climbing caseload, Project Straighttalk targeted three predominantly black neighborhoods where high-risk drug use proliferated. Project staff "saturate[d] the high-risk target communities with AIDS risk-reduction information," taking bleach kits, AIDS pamphlets, and needle-sterilization guidelines door to door in those communities.[72] Workers also took their message to prisons, soup kitchens, detox centers, homeless shelters, and "shooting galleries" throughout the county. The state AIDS Control Branch also funded similar harm-reduction programs in Fayetteville and Winston-Salem, but Durham County's program proved the most innovative. African Americans had finally begun hearing AIDS messages specifically targeted to them from both state and local health educators.

AS 1988 DREW TO A CLOSE, Harold Burton grew so sick that he could no longer work, and neither could he maintain his AIDS education efforts. He could not pay his rent, he had no insurance to afford AZT, and he was too sick to qualify for a clinical trial. Ultimately he moved in with his sister Louise, but he quickly grew so ill that she had to readmit him to the hospital. In April, Burton died.[73] For Louise Alston, her brother's death proved a new beginning: she had worked informally alongside Burton for over two years, warning drug users not to share needles. Seeing her brother's rapid demise, remembering his poor treatment, and recognizing the disproportionate impact AIDS was having on black men prompted Alston to offer to work with Howard Fitts at the Durham Committee AIDS program, and within weeks, she started work.[74]

BY 1989, NORTH CAROLINA was devoting greater attention to AIDS: private citizens, politicians, and advocacy groups mobilized to grapple with the disease. White gay men showed the most progress, marshaling private capital and public resources to create an AIDS infrastructure across the state and a strong policy alliance in the capitol. Education and experience put men like David Jolly and David Jones in strategic positions to influence AIDS policy. African Americans, the other group most affected by the epidemic, had much further to go: few had mobilized around AIDS and even fewer and leveraged political capital to deal with AIDS in minority communities. The people making public demands and guiding AIDS policy in North Carolina were not black.

Access to services unfolded in a much similar way. White gay men had developed many of the AIDS services in the state, and the mainstream gay community mobilized to take advantage of them. In cities like Raleigh, Durham, and Charlotte, gay men had embraced those affected by AIDS, identifying with them, publicizing their predicament, and designing prevention programs that took their cultural needs into consideration. Early on, MAP's controversial safer sex cards symbolized the way gay men had integrated AIDS harm reduction into everyday gay life.

The African American experience could not have been more different. African Americans with AIDS did not learn of, or did not take advantage of, the services offered by AIDS organizations until well into the decade, despite the fact that they had acquired the disease in roughly equivalent numbers from the outset. This meant black families, like Louise Alston's, bore the brunt of care for black patients with AIDS when many were not in the financial position to do so. Moreover, the African American community did not embrace those with AIDS nor publicize their plight. The discomfort many felt about the modes of transmission and the near ubiquity of white gay leadership in the AIDS fight meant that few black churches and civic groups focused on the problem and few African Americans volunteered with AIDS organizations. Since many still saw AIDS as a disease of white gays, and since sexual relationships between black and white have had a long and complicated history in American society, it was difficult for established AIDS advocacy groups to develop culturally competent safer sex messages. So AIDS existed in the silences. Black families like Harold Burton's lied about the disease that claimed their child's life, while many black gays lied to themselves about their risks and to others about how they had acquired the disease.[75]

Meanwhile, North Carolina's political will on AIDS stood at cross-purposes with the most pressing aspects of its epidemic: the continued spread of AIDS into African American communities. By 1989, data suggested that AIDS rates had plateaued among white gay men but continued to rise in every category among African Americans. These trends garnered only moderate attention in the policy arena, while the clash between white gay men and social conservatives consumed tremendous energy and attention.[76] For their part, conservatives called for traditional testing and surveillance methods, but, in their repulsion toward homosexuality and drug use, they resisted confidence-building measures that would have protected the lives and livelihoods of gay men and induce them to cooperate. Gay men—black and white alike—had a long history of reasons to suspect that social conservatives would not protect their privacy, and, consequently, they opposed traditional public health measures in favor of voluntary and anonymous testing and outreach measures. While these educational programs worked within white gay culture, they proved largely ineffective in black gay culture. Black gays remained largely impervious to AIDS prevention efforts at the end of the 1980s.

Health officials and AIDS organizations failed to recognize this problem.

Gay organizations like the LGHP assumed an affinity between white and black gays and underestimated the ethnocultural differences that might hinder outreach efforts. Black organizations like Howard Fitts's AIDS Clearinghouse presumed solidarity between gay and straight blacks and misjudged the pervasive homophobia in black communities. Both groups failed in their efforts to reach black gays. Moreover, neither group understood the unique context of AIDS in black communities. White gays worked hard to ameliorate the financial consequences of AIDS but knew little about the economic context that put African Americans at greater risk for HIV/AIDS from the outset. Conversely, put off as they were by what they considered the stains of immorality and addiction, black community leaders failed to see how black HIV rates fit into the larger context of poverty and structural discrimination. State and local health workers also lacked the cultural competence to reach these high-risk communities. Thus at the end of the 1980s, when white gay communities were beginning to see positive AIDS data and experience political success, North Carolina's AIDS epidemic continued to ravish the high-risk minority communities least able to defend themselves.[77]

CHAPTER 4

BLACK MEN DIE A THOUSAND DIFFERENT WAYS

AIDS in African American Communities

Sometime in the late 1980s, Garry Lipscomb of the Lesbian and Gay Health Project (LGHP) attended a meeting at Mt. Olive Baptist Church in northern Durham County. "They wanted to talk about the AIDS epidemic," Lipscomb remembered, "and they had people, mostly drug users, who were talking about getting infected and turning around and how this was really a good thing for them that they had gotten this and they were living better lives." Lipscomb found this emphasis somewhat troubling, particularly in light of the dramatic rise of HIV in black communities. So, when it was his turn to speak, Lipscomb posed a direct challenge to the gathered congregants. "I got up and spoke about needing volunteers to get out there and work with someone who had HIV," Lipscomb recalled. "They didn't want to hear that there was a need for them to actually go and work with people that they didn't know who had AIDS."[1]

It was in this context that Lipscomb encountered Howard Fitts. "When he got involved, there were much more middle-class folks who starting seeing that there was a need to do things differently," Lipscomb noted. "A couple of the churches started doing things. . . . He put respectability on it, it was okay for other people to talk about it." Unfortunately, Lipscomb pointed out, there were not enough people like Fitts: "It would have made a difference, but there just weren't."[2]

While it was profoundly valuable for black organizations to join the fight against HIV/AIDS, it was not clear how effective these groups were at addressing HIV/AIDS in African American communities. Challenges on several different levels—structural, institutional, cultural, and organizational—all conspired to hamper outreach efforts while contributing to the spread of the virus in vulnerable minority communities. This chapter explores the nature of these challenges and the role they had in the limited effectiveness of AIDS programs among African Americans in North Carolina.

HOWARD FITTS'S AIDS CLEARINGHOUSE symbolized the larger commitment that North Carolina had made to funding AIDS Service Organizations in African American communities. Community-based AIDS organizations had been a passion of David Jolly's even before he became head of the state's AIDS program, and soon after Jolly arrived at the state health department, he and Rebecca Meriwether determined to obtain as much money as they could from the Centers for Disease Control and Prevention (CDC) for community groups. "We knew we couldn't do what needed to be done at the grassroots level from the state," David Jolly later explained. "So we set up a grant process and funded a lot of projects."[3] Standard programs like the Metrolina AIDS Project (MAP) and the LGHP received funding, but Jolly also worked hard to get support for programs targeting minority communities like Teens Against AIDS (a Raleigh program coordinated by Strengthening the Black Family), Project First Step (a Winston-Salem substance abuse program), and the Minority AIDS Project in Rocky Mount (run by the local Opportunities Industrialization Center). Other programs, like Cumberland County's Minority AIDS Speakers Bureau (launched in 1991) received state support to bring AIDS awareness to black congregations on their annual "AIDS Sunday."[4]

This state support notwithstanding, providing adequate AIDS education for minorities in a multicounty region proved a daunting task for groups like the AIDS Clearinghouse. Few of the county health departments offered AIDS education and prevention programs at all, much less for high-risk minority groups.[5] With few black men as health educators and few culturally competent AIDS materials and prevention strategies, Fitts and his team worried that most AIDS warnings held little relevance for black men who had sex with men.[6] After about six months, Fitts and his team had made little headway "identify[ing] groups of black homosexual males" with which to partner in their efforts against AIDS.[7] Worried that their efforts to reach high-risk individuals would continue to prove ineffective and hoping to maximize their limited resources, Fitts and his team expanded their efforts to black communities by taking their message to black churches, colleges, NAACP chapters, and medical professionals.[8] Fitts and his team hoped this scattershot approach would raise general community awareness about AIDS while also taking advantage of "the presence of homosexuals in any groups where presentations [were] being made."[9] They also trusted that black men who have sex with men (MSM) would be able to find adequate information on AIDS from the larger gay community. In the meantime, the AIDS Clearinghouse worked to reach as many people as possible.

The immense needs and limited resources that the AIDS Clearinghouse found in its region were echoed in numerous communities across the state. To address these growing problems, North Carolinians exerted an immense collective investment in its AIDS infrastructure in the late 1980s, as community groups and government officials sought to stem the tide of the epidemic. One key area of concern was AIDS housing. In Charlotte, activists founded the Brothers Foundation in the summer of 1989 to "open a group home for low-income AIDS patients" who had lost most other affordable housing options.[10] That same summer, Durham's AIDS Community Residence Association (ACRA) opened the state's first AIDS-care facility, and Wake County advocates opened the second AIDS-care facility, Hustead House, a year later.[11] Religious groups in the state also began launching AIDS programs. By 1990, so many denominations had started some sort of AIDS effort that the North Carolina Council of Churches created a task force on AIDS to coordinate the efforts, reduce duplication of services, and enable smaller churches to start new ministries in their regions.[12] The following year, Southern Baptist pastor Deborah Warren created the Regional AIDS Interfaith Network (RAIN) in Charlotte to coordinate volunteer efforts between Christian and non-Christian faith communities so that members of multiple congregations could visit people with AIDS, provide them transportation, complete household tasks, and take them to community events.[13] Soon thereafter, similar church-affiliated networks sprang up in Guilford County (Guilford Regional AIDS Interfaith Network) and the Triangle area (Triangle AIDS Interfaith Network).

Other groups flourished, too, like those in rural areas and those specializing in AIDS programs for women and minorities. In rural Morganton, the AIDS Leadership Foothills Alliance was providing support groups, AIDS buddies, referral services, a speakers' bureau, and a resource library to over thirty people with AIDS in six counties.[14] In Robeson County, health workers noticed alarming spikes in HIV rates among minority women and adolescents and secured a three-year grant to get AIDS information to American Indian and African American women and teens.[15] In Charlotte, the rising number of heterosexual — particularly female — clients forced MAP to craft programs geared specifically toward women and poorer families (in 1991 over 60 percent of MAP's new clients were heterosexual, and 65 percent seeking information were women).[16] MAP launched a Women and AIDS Coalition and began providing clients with transportation, emergency funds, financial support, food and medical supplies, and Social Security application assistance.[17]

As service groups proliferated, they began coordinating services. In January 1990, representatives from Mecklenburg and six other counties met to launch the Regional HIV Consortium, the result of one of twenty-two federal grants enabling regional plans for comprehensive AIDS services that shared programs and consolidated efforts.[18] Their $147,000 grant funded awareness-raising, stigma-reduction, and volunteer training for physicians, morticians, and faith- and community-based AIDS care groups.[19] One month later, North Carolina's Department of Environment, Health, and Natural Resources met to create similar consortia in eight other areas of the state.[20] AIDS Service Organizations or AIDS task forces in each region joined forces with county or regional mental health agencies, social services groups, health centers, substance abuse centers, and hospices to craft more seamless and comprehensive health and support service delivery.[21] Four of the state's earliest AIDS organizations—the LGHP in Durham, MAP in Charlotte, GROW in Wilmington, and the Western North Carolina AIDS Project in Asheville—became lead organizations in North Carolina's consortium plan.

These moves positioned North Carolina to benefit from the Ryan White Comprehensive AIDS Resources Emergency (CARE) Act, which Congress passed in 1990. The program promised to fill gaps in the state's AIDS delivery system. North Carolina already ranked in the top twenty states in terms of residents diagnosed with HIV/AIDS, and since it accounted for more than 1 percent of national cases in the nation, it was well on its way to being designated a "moderate incident state" by the federal government (this officially occurred in 1991).[22] The funds allowed an even greater improvement in AIDS services provided to minorities. In February 1991, for example, the Durham County Health Department opened an early intervention HIV clinic in a high-risk and historically black part of Durham.[23] The clinic—the first of its kind in the state—managed HIV infection in patients before their disease grew critical and ensured that patients who previously lacked comprehensive coverage received continuity of care.[24]

Improving the state's response to HIV was necessary because HIV was spreading aggressively, particularly among blacks. Infections among African Americans continued climbing well into the early 1990s (see fig. 4.1). The circle of those infected also continued to expand: while MSM and male intravenous drug users made up the bulk of the disease burden in African American communities (each accounted for between 20 and 30 percent of cases), heterosexuals, female drug users, and other at-risk populations accounted for an additional 5 to 10 percent each. Between 1981 and 1996, 86 percent of women, 66 percent of adolescents (aged thirteen to nineteen), and 81 percent of children (infant to age twelve) infected with the disease were African

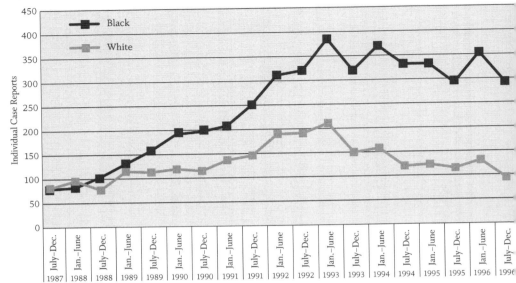

FIGURE 4.1. North Carolina HIV/AIDS Cases by Race, 1987–1996

Source: U.S. Department of Health and Human Services, Centers for Disease Control and Prevention, National Center for HIV, STD and TB Prevention, AIDS Public Information Data Set, U.S. Surveillance Data for 1981–2002, CDC WONDER Downloadable Database, software version 2.7.1, December 2005.

American.[25] HIV directly affected a diverse and continually diversifying set of populations within black communities, and health workers struggled to keep up.

These two trends—the expansion of the AIDS service infrastructure in North Carolina and the ongoing and disproportionate spread of HIV among African Americans in the state—prompted several questions: what factors were driving the epidemic in African American communities, what elements influenced the shape of the response policy, and how effective were those efforts to address the problem?

As mentioned in chapter 1, several population-level risks made members of African American communities more vulnerable to HIV infection, and many of these contributed to the spread of HIV in North Carolina. Individual choices, group behaviors, social structures, and historical influences formed a complex nexus of risk.[26] Several individual factors make people more vulnerable to sexually transmitted infections, including negative influences (like drug use, peer risk behavior, history of sexual abuse, and experience with risky sexual behaviors) and a low level of positive influences (including religiosity, self-efficacy, family stability, and personal ambition).[27] Numerous structural factors in the state appear to have put African Americans at greater risk for these individual risks, including poverty, substance abuse, insufficient access to medical care, incarceration policy and patterns, short- and long-term migration trends, and the nature of heterosexual and homosexual sexual networks.

Perhaps the most obvious structural factor rendering African American communities vulnerable to HIV was poverty and its associated problems. Poverty did not cause HIV/AIDS, of course, but it did increase the number of social and medical vulnerabilities in a person's life. The high rates of unemployment and long-term joblessness in many of North Carolina's African American communities permitted drug economies to flourish in some neighborhoods, making needle- and addiction-associated transmission more possible.[28] Poverty also pushed some individuals into survival sex. AIDS specialist Charles van der Horst recalled:

> When I first came [to UNC] in '88 there was a black medical student who wanted to work with me, and I said, "You know, I have no idea who these people are, these new patients who are starting to come. I want you to just interview twenty black people, half women, half men, and just find out who they are, where they were born, where they grew up, who they live with, how they earn their money. What do they do for their day? How do they think they got infected?" And of them, four people were actively prostituting and prostituting just to pay their heating bill that winter. He was interviewing in the winter. And they were going to Raleigh to have sex, anonymous sex as prostitutes. So that was just a horrifying thing to me, both for them personally, that someone would have to prostitute themselves in order to pay their bills, and that the epidemic was never going to end.[29]

Poverty also hampered medical access. African Americans in North Carolina—particularly black women—were less able to afford primary care than Caucasians, and primary care physicians had few financial incentives to practice in black communities.[30] Historical mistrust of the (largely white) medical establishment also kept many African Americans from seeking treatment until the disease became critical, even among those who possessed medical insurance.[31] Danny Moore, a black man from Fayetteville, for example, was diagnosed with AIDS in 1987. He initially feared revealing his diagnosis to his family because three of his brothers had already died from disease or violence. "Black men die a thousand different ways," Moore's mother responded with resignation when he finally broke the news to her. "It could have been cancer or any other disease."[32] Moore's lack of insurance kept him from getting an HIV test until it was clear he was sick, and it meant he could not afford the new antivirals (AZT) that had become available for people with AIDS that year. It was not until the summer of 1988, when he was enrolled in a clinical trial at Duke University, that he was able to get the drug.[33] Harold Burton, discussed in chapter 3, likewise was trapped at the intersection of AIDS, poverty, and poor health: by late 1988 he had grown so sick that he could no longer continue to work or continue his AIDS volunteer activities. Without employment, Burton lost his housing, his health insurance, and his access to AZT. He was too sick to qualify for any clinical trials. Ultimately, in his final months, Burton had to depend on his sister and the safety-net health care system to provide him with end-of-life care.[34]

Even black patients visiting black doctors suffered access issues since, according to one report, most black doctors were "not affiliated with a major medical university and thus not acquainted with the latest treatments for AIDS and not easily able to access experimental AIDS drugs," and AIDS research at the time routinely excluded women and minorities.[35] So as new AIDS therapies and improved prognoses emerged, high drug costs often made treatment prohibitive for poor people. "[We are trying] to get people into the experimental things," Fred McCree of Wilmington's AIDS Awareness in the Black Community Project (AABC), explained in early 1990. "Treatment will get more expensive and more out of reach for poor people. Poor people are going to have to have more advocates."[36]

At the state level, however, most AIDS workers still missed the connection between AIDS and poverty: "I don't remember people talking about the relationship between poverty and health," David Jolly said about his years running the state AIDS program. "We were working long days, you know 10 to 12 hour days, and I . . . didn't have the time to read about it."[37] Under the radar of most health workers, AIDS increasingly became tied to the lives of poor people in North Carolina.

Harold Burton's experience highlights a second structural factor making African Americans more vulnerable to the spread of HIV in North Carolina: Drug use directly (through contaminated needles) and indirectly (through the amplification of risky behavior and the exchange of sex for drugs) contributed to the spread of AIDS in African American communities.[38] The supply of inexpensive drugs—both cocaine and heroin—flooded North Carolina cities like Fayetteville and Durham from Asia and Latin America in the mid- to late 1980s, and drug use disproportionately affected impoverished black communities.[39] Ninety percent of injection drug users shared needles, and a considerable number maintained sexual relationships with nonusing partners. Consequently, between 1985 and 1987, HIV infection among drug users rose 500 percent, and among heterosexuals it rose 600 percent. Drugs played a disproportionate role in the spread of AIDS among African Americans in the state: 90 percent of drug users with HIV/AIDS and 90 percent of heterosexuals with the disease were African American, and, where statistics were available, most of those who acquired HIV heterosexually (90 percent of black women and 70 percent of black men) acquired it from a drug-using partner.[40] By the late 1980s, blacks acquired HIV more through drug use than through any other means.[41] These trends continued into the 1990s, as cocaine and crack cocaine continued flowing out of Miami and New York along major highways into North Carolina cities.[42] Powdered cocaine flooded the market at bargain prices, and chips of crack sold for as little as ten dollars apiece across the state.[43] Poor drug users who were willing to exchange sex for drugs became especially vulnerable, mainly because they tended not to perceive their risk or to use condoms, and black women were disproportionately represented in this population.[44] The state and local communities were cognizant of these problems and had taken steps to address them—most notably in Durham, where the Health Department was distributing needle-cleaning kits in high-risk communities in the city—but the expanding market of inexpensive drugs easily outstripped their best efforts.[45] As the epidemic moved into its second decade, the problem of drug-related HIV transmission in minority communities accelerated.

The particular shape of heterosexual sexual networks within African American communities further compounded the vulnerabilities brought about by poverty and substance abuse. Drug-related HIV transmission appears to have been a key driver of the epidemic.[46] Once the virus entered heterosexual sexual networks, two other factors appear to have come into play. First, North Carolina sexual networks were profoundly segregated by race: most African Americans in the state had sexual relationships with other African Americans; most Caucasians had sex with other Caucasians. This created "highly interconnected [sexual] networks with potential for rapid propagation of HIV and other STIs."[47] Second, some subgroups within African American communities in North Carolina had higher rates of sexual concurrency (overlapping or simultaneous sexual partnerships) than the population as a whole.[48] Indeed, since blacks were more likely than whites or Hispanics to have sexual partners who themselves had had at least four other partners in the previous year, even blacks with a low number of sexual partners stood at greater risk than whites of acquiring HIV and other STIs.[49] Sexual concurrency on its own facilitated viral spread within African American communities, and when combined with the segregated nature of sexual networks in the state, it made African American communities particularly vulnerable to rapid heterosexual HIV transmission.

Incarceration also continued to contribute to HIV's spread in African American communities. As mentioned in chapter 1, North Carolina disproportionately incarcerated African Americans, and by the late 1980s incarceration rates were widely divergent when analyzed by race. A key factor driving these divergent rates came from North Carolina's "tough on crime" stance toward drug-related crimes: between 1984 and 1994, drug-related crimes soared in North Carolina, and the incarceration rate followed suit.[50] In 1992, criminal justice scholar Stephens Clarke noted that drug arrests of minorities in the state climbed five times faster than those of whites between 1984 and 1989: from 5,021 arrests to 14,192 for minorities (a 183 percent increase), and from 10,269 to 14,007 for whites (a 36 percent increase).[51] These trends only compounded the role incarceration played in the spread of HIV. Prisons became repositories for people in the drug economy, that is, those who engaged in drug and sexual activities conducive to the spread of HIV both in jail and upon release.[52] High incarceration rates, in turn, intensified the social disruption experienced by the communities from which these (disproportionately) young men were extracted: women and dependent children experienced deeper socioeconomic insecurity, and separational concurrency became even more likely.[53]

The connection between AIDS and prison had been seen in the state since at least 1983, when the first reports of infected prisoners emerged. By the end of the decade, sixty-two inmates had developed AIDS (one-third were released, and one-half had already died).[54] Prison officials had initially responded slowly to the problem, and by the time they awakened to the crisis, the state had implemented its anonymous testing regime, which barred officials from mandatory testing. The rising number of affected prisoners, along with the promise of new therapies, prompted officials to call for a new policy in the spring of 1989. That May, lawmakers floated a bill providing "for detection, prevention and treatment of AIDS in prison."[55] The bill allowed for HIV testing in prisons so corrections officials could assess the scope of the problem and plan accordingly.[56] As soon as the bill passed in early November, prison officials began testing new inmates.[57] Within six months, preliminary data showed that 3.1 percent of new inmates were infected, above the national average for prisons and well above the state average for infection rates.[58] "The prison system is becoming a repository for indigent people infected with HIV," the Correction Department's health services director concluded.[59] Consequently, corrections officials sought $7 million from lawmakers to improve AIDS care and prevention in state prisons.[60]

News about AIDS in North Carolina prisons worried AIDS activists like Howard Fitts. Concerned that blacks would face the worst of it, Fitts charged Louise Alston with the task of AIDS education in prisons. "Dr. Fitts said, 'This is one of the things I would like . . . to go into,'" Alston recalled. "Well I said, 'That's fantastic. . . . That's what I would like to do Dr. Fitts.' So we starting going around to the different cities, talking to the people who were a head of the prison system or the jails and say, 'We would like to come in and do education.' And they gave us permission. And I went once a month to all these places. Everyday I was going to somebody's prison, somebody's jail, talking to them . . . to do the AIDS education."[61]

Most corrections officials appreciated this work, but not all. "We had a . . . sheriff down in Halifax County," Howard Fitts remembered. "I had approached him. He said, 'I'm not gonna have a woman goin' in my jail talkin' about. . . .' It was like a real reaction: that was not a consideration he even approved."[62] Except in Halifax County, Louise Alston became the primary AIDS educator for inmates in the Piedmont.

In addition to incarceration policies and patterns, both long- and short-term migration patterns continued to make African American communities vulnerable to HIV. Long-term migratory forces appear to have affected the whole state, while seasonal migration signaled the growing threat HIV/AIDS posed to rural areas. The Great Migration (between 1890 and 1970) had pushed six million blacks — disproportionately men — out of the American South.[63] Then, the Great Return Migration drew millions of African Americans back into the South after 1970; in the latter half of the 1970s alone, 14,456 blacks moved to the state; between 1985 and 1990, that number jumped to 39,015.[64] A large number of these new migrants were young, single, unemployed black women, and they moved to North Carolina's cities (Raleigh-Durham proved most popular).[65] Thus, by 1990, African Americans in North Carolina had a general sex ratio of 0.88; for black women between the ages of twenty-five and forty-four, the ratio dropped to 0.86, and for women in their thirties, the number dropped to 0.84.[66] Migration continued skewing gender ratios which, in turn, created an environment conducive to HIV transmission. The relative scarcity of black men put some black women at a relational disadvantage in their communities. Some demanded less of their partners (like condom use or monogamous relationships) to remain financially or socially secure.[67] Consequently, the rate of female-headed households rose and the rate of sexual concurrency in parts of the black community soared, creating a fertile environment for HIV transmission.[68] Unsurprisingly, cases of heterosexually acquired HIV mushroomed in North Carolina, and black women constituted the bulk of them.

Seasonal migrants had been one of the first groups indicating the disproportionate spread of HIV in African American communities. The North Carolina economy depends on migrant farmworkers to harvest its crops, so thousands of migrant farmers — mostly blacks and Hispanics — come to the state each year to pick apples or tobacco before trekking southward to Florida. These workers have little access to health care, suffer poor health, and experience profound social instability.[69] In the fall of 1987, a study of one group of farmworkers indicated that HIV was profoundly affecting black seasonal workers.[70] Indeed, only the black farmworkers in the cohort tested positive for HIV: the rate of HIV infection among black males was 5.9 percent; the rate among black females was 2.3 percent; and the HIV rates among individuals who reported having syphilis were double the rates of those without it (5.6 percent and 2.2 percent, respectively). The strongly segregated nature of the study data suggested that HIV/AIDS would disproportionately affect African Americans in rural North Carolina as well.[71]

One final, essential structural component increasing the spread of HIV in North Carolina was the role of black MSM. The relation of these men both to African American communities and to gay communities was particularly complex, and it had a profound impact on the HIV risk among these men. According to Carlton Rutherford, a gay black man from North Carolina who was diagnosed with AIDS in 1986, black MSM lived from birth "separated from mainstream America," which meant their primary support came "from the black community, not the gay community."[72] However, in many cases, homophobia within the black community created a double separation.[73] Rutherford explained the dilemma: "[Black pastors] get up in church and say 'You're going to hell' . . . [so] why would you come out and say that you're sick? Then they'll say it's because you're gay that you got AIDS. . . . Then people reject you. . . . Coming out doesn't happen."[74]

In addition to their contested relationship with the larger black community, black MSM had an uncertain relationship with the larger gay community. In the first place, for many, the terms "gay" and "gay community" did not fit, that is, they did not consider themselves gay and/or part of a "gay community." In addition, many of the black men who did self-identify as gay did not see themselves as part of the larger gay movement because, led as it was by white gay men, they believed it to be unconcerned about the black freedom struggle.[75] Majority gay culture was irrelevant to their experience. Consequently, in North Carolina, black MSM created autonomous subcultures that rarely overlapped with white gay institutions or organizations. These included informal leisure societies and private social clubs, with individuals permitted entry only by invitation or word of mouth; and white gay men were largely unwelcome.[76]

Black MSM's marginalization by both the black community and the white gay community had troubling consequences. First, racially segregated homosexual networks gave many black men a false sense of security. "They really believed [AIDS was a disease of] white men, and most of these guys . . . did not have sex with white men," explained Garry Lipscomb, an AIDS educator with LGHP.[77] Second, the hidden nature of North Carolina's black gay infrastructure diminished the ability of grassroots prevention efforts to combat riskier sex practices or raise the specter of risk.[78] "[Everybody was saying,] 'Let's have a lot of sex,'" Lipscomb said of North Carolina's black gay sexual culture of the early 1990s. "I think people knew that they were putting themselves at risk, but . . . the majority of people I talked to really honestly did not think that they were going to get infected."[79] The misperception of risk and barriers to external prevention efforts combined with the sexual segregation and the risky sexual behavior to facilitate rapid viral transmission within black gay sexual networks.

On top of these structural factors, several institutional factors worked against a robust effort to address HIV/AIDS in the African American community. Some of these included poor coordination of care efforts, ideology-based policy disagreements, institutional limitations at the state level, and underrepresentation of minorities in mainstream AIDS groups. None of these factors can directly be implicated in the spread of HIV in African American communities, but each were part of a larger policy environment in which minority AIDS received inadequate attention and resources from policymakers, health workers, and community members.

Coordination of AIDS care and prevention proved difficult in many parts of North Carolina because communities often lacked the resources or a "lead organization" to address AIDS. As mentioned above, some communities—like Mecklenburg County and the surrounding regions—recognized these problems in the late 1980s and sought federal funding to coordinate their regional care infrastructure.[80] Many communities lacked organizational cohesion or a central organization that could lead the AIDS care and control efforts, and in some cases, the state-sponsored consortia plan that came in 1990 merely papered over these community deficits.[81]

Durham County served as one example of these organizational problems. The LGHP had played an important role in the origins and development of North Carolina's AIDS response. As more and varied community groups entered the AIDS arena in the latter 1980s, however, LGHP was forced to wrestle with its identity in the AIDS community alongside church groups, housing advocates, and service organizations. As more groups contended for public and nonprofit funds, some board members felt the LGHP's gay identity and nontraditional organizational structure put it at a competitive disadvantage for this funding. Consequently, the project restructured its leadership from a steering committee to a board and created a semiseparate entity called The AIDS Service Project (TASP) in 1988 to make the organization more recognizable and acceptable to foundations and government agencies.[82] The LGHP had not restructured quickly enough, however, and by early 1989 — after several grant applications failed and some fund-raisers flopped — the LGHP found itself on shaky financial footing.[83] A leadership controversy ensued, as the financial insecurities exposed a growing level of dissatisfaction over the organization's leadership and direction.[84] Jill Duvall, the director at the time, came under fire from some LGHP supporters for her radical feminist politics, but, more importantly, they questioned her and LGHP's effectiveness in tackling the problem of AIDS in the local community.[85] Tony Adinolfi, an LGHP board member and the support-group administrator at the Duke AIDS Clinic, was quite vocal about this latter concern. "I remember in the annual report of the Health Project that said they had given service to 'blank' amount of people," he said. "So I just asked them who are those people? . . . I never got an answer as to where those people were."[86] From the state's perspective, these general numbers were enough. "LGHP really flourished for awhile under Jill Duvall's leadership," David Jolly remembered.[87] "I'd say that was the most successful period of the Health Project. It was at its apex under Jill's reign; it was financially stable; it was well respected; it was a pretty well-oiled machine. Jill was good."[88] The actual caregivers doubted these figures, however. "We [were] supposed to be giving services to people," Adinolfi recalled. "We should have [the numbers] broken down [by] where these people [were] so when we ask[ed] for more money later, they'll [ask] where are the people you provided service for? I never got an answer. So I . . . felt that those numbers were made up, because if I didn't know . . . I was in the [AIDS] clinic everyday of my life, I never saw people from the Health Project there."[89] Looking back, Duvall acknowledged that the numbers sometimes lacked formal consistency, but she maintained that neither she nor any other staff intentionally ignored a board request, arguing that conflict really centered on whether she or the board wielded power in the organization.[90]

Regardless of the cause of the conflict, the quarrel hurt LGHP's credibility.[91] Many middle-class gays and lesbians began supporting other, less controversial, AIDS programs, like ACRA, Meals on Wheels, or the AIDS Services Agency in Raleigh.[92] Moreover, local AIDS clinics started their own AIDS services or referred clients to other, more reliable organizations. Tony Adinolfi at Duke sent people with AIDS to Greensboro's Triad Health Project, Raleigh's AIDS Services Agency, or a group of Triangle churches that soon coalesced into the Triangle AIDS Interfaith Network (TRAIN).[93] The controversy ended LGHP's tenure as the preferred AIDS service provider in the region, squandering LGHP's strategic position in the Triangle and opening the door for other organizations to compete for clients and, ultimately, financial resources. It also meant that, when the state later opted to establish LGHP as the lead organization in the Regional AIDS Consortium, it proved unable to turn that authority into effective AIDS care and prevention.

Having a coordinated institutional response in a region did not ensure that the needs of minority communities were adequately addressed, however. In the late 1980s and early 1990s, most mainstream AIDS organizations in the state lacked racial diversity within their leadership and had few mechanisms to address minority AIDS concerns. For example, the LGHP had only two African Americans on its board, a black lesbian (Brenda Edwards) and a black gay man (Godfrey Herndon), and only one black man (Garry Lipscomb) serving as a buddy for other black men.[94] The AIDS Services Agency of Wake County (ASA) likewise struggled to recruit black volunteers for its growing number of minority clients. Only 20 of its 200 volunteers were black, and only 2 of the group's 48 AIDS "buddies" were black.[95] Metrolina AIDS Project, in Charlotte, had similar problems.[96] Moreover, the state's AIDS lobbying group, the NC AIDS Service Coalition, listed no black AIDS organizations among its constituents in the late 1980s, despite the existence of at least five state-supported groups in the state.[97]

What drove this underrepresentation? "Part of the problem is that our other programs have not reached out to the black community, part of it is probably a lack of awareness among blacks about the nature and extent of the illness," ASA director Cullen Gurganus told reporters in 1991. "Whatever the reasons, we need to recruit more people of color."[98] On the ground, some white volunteers blamed blacks for the underrepresentation. "It irritates the livin' devil out of me," one white volunteer told reporters. "The gay commu-

nity is now taking care of the black community. Nobody took care of gays—
we had to take care of our own. This woman I was driving [to an AIDS clinic]
knew so little about AIDS. Where are the blacks?"[99] "We would love to see
more black involvement," ASA's Jacquelyn Clymore acknowledged to reporters, "but so far we haven't had much luck."[100]

Indeed, some observers worried that concern over AIDS would wane as
the disease grew more manageable and gay activists obtained their policy
demands. "When the image of AIDS was as a white, gay disease, it had the
advantages of the activism and social power that the gay community brought
to it," Herbert Nickens, vice president for minority health at the American
Association of Medical Colleges, told reporters in 1991. "But as it gets perceived as a minority disease, this will change. Minority diseases, particularly
those of IV drug users and their sexual partners and children, do not have
great power in society. . . . The real danger is that this could be labeled as a
disease of people who are expendable."[101]

Garry Lipscomb tried bridging the divide between black and white gays,
but many African Americans treated him as if he had chosen the white community over them. "I did kind of feel like an outsider," Lipscomb recalled.
"But I never lost that connection. I was always trying to stay in there."[102]
Because he was black, the LGHP relied heavily on him to partner with its
black clients with AIDS. "I worked with two or three guys at the same time
because there was nobody else," Lipscomb explained. This ultimately gave
Lipscomb access to a very closeted pocket of black gays in Durham. "There
was one guy I stayed with [as a buddy] for like two years," Lipscomb recalled.
". . . They called him "Blue" . . . partly because he drove a blue Riveria. . . . He
was this big, dark-skinned black man. And of course he was not out—nobody
knew he was gay. And he was the one who introduced me to the people at the
Stable [a private, invitation-only social club for black gays in Durham] . . .
and that was a great introduction for me because at that point . . . [AIDS was]
really affecting our community and no one was doing anything."[103]

One obvious solution to the problem of reaching out to at-risk African
Americans, then, was to rely on AIDS programs headed by African Americans.
In the late 1980s, several were established across the state. In Charlotte (and
several other southern cities), the Southern Christian Leadership Conference
used a $1.5 million federal grant to start AIDS programs in local schools.[104]
In Wilmington, the organization AIDS Awareness in the Black Community
began training black churches to address the epidemic. And in the Piedmont,
the Durham Committee's AIDS Clearinghouse worked to overcome the

"extremely limited . . . AIDS outreach" available to local blacks by expanding its focus from the "difficult to reach" to "minority populations in general."[105] Howard Fitts and his team continued taking their AIDS message to school administrators, black churches, county task forces, youth groups, NAACP chapters, and black community leaders.[106]

Despite this spike in organizing, black AIDS groups remained a minority within the constellation of AIDS organizations. While the state encouraged minority groups to collaborate with one other to multiply their effect, they offered relatively limited funds for minority projects. In 1989, for example, the state renewed Howard Fitts's AIDS funding with the stipulation that his AIDS Clearinghouse begin working with a newly founded minority AIDS group in Rocky Mount that the state was now funding.[107] The AIDS Clearinghouse did collaborate with the group, but within two years, Fitts and his team found themselves competing with this same group for state funds.

At the state level, several barriers made reaching African Americans more difficult. The first was merely a staffing question: who should the state hire to respond best to the growing epidemic? Between 1988 and 1990, blacks went from 52 to 64 percent of all AIDS cases in the state. During that time, the state hired several African American health educators to run AIDS education programs and several more to notify partners of people with HIV.[108] Still, by 1990, less than 40 percent of AIDS intervention specialists in North Carolina were African American.[109] David Jolly later acknowledged, "We were getting it, because we realized we needed to be hiring African American people, [but] I am sure that we could have done a much better job."[110] Even here, however, there were difficulties: almost all the new health educators hired by the state were black women.[111] "We would have been delighted to hire an African American male," David Jolly recalled, "[but] there [were] no black men who [were] health educators."[112] Indeed, in 1990, black men accounted for less than 10 percent of the AIDS program staff.[113] With men constituting over two-thirds of HIV cases among African Americans in the state, the scarcity of male health educators robbed the state's outreach program of whatever insights they might have brought to effective interventions.

Resistance from social conservatives also slowed state efforts to be culturally competent. "I spent 85 percent of my time trying to prevent bad things from happening within our own administration!" Jolly recalled. "I mean, we had very little time and energy left to do the positive stuff. We were just constantly trying to hold back the tide against these Neanderthals."[114] He also recalled that at least one high-ranking official in the governor's administration considered AIDS "a solution" rather than "a problem," and that other prominent staff in the health division were quite vocal about their disinterest in working with "these AIDS people."[115] In addition, the state's public relations department frequently tried to censor Jolly's educational material.[116] In one case, state officials seized 25,000 copies of a Spanish-language brochure after Jolly's team failed to get proper approval of the translation.[117] Since the brochure illustrated how to put a condom on an erect penis, Jolly and his team feared the move was merely a pretext to seize the English version as well, so he and his staff smuggled 950,000 copies of the English version out of the office, hiding them in the homes of local AIDS activists. The following day, administration officials demanded Jolly's team remove depictions of pubic hair from the pictures in the Spanish-language brochures. When Jolly pointed out that doing so would make the pictures look like pre-adolescent boys, the officials immediately reconsidered, permitting the use of pubic hair in the pictures but insisting that number of pictures be reduced from three to two. The administration took no action on the (now hidden) English brochures and Jolly's team reprinted the Spanish brochures. Periodically thereafter, an administration watchdog would appear at Jolly's AIDS control office and search the files for materials that "encouraged homosexuality." Since the office usually received one day's notice about an administrator's visit, Jolly and his staff always removed any potentially controversial material the night before, and the administration seized no other AIDS documents. Nevertheless, Jolly's team felt besieged, and Jolly personally felt "written off" as "the loudmouth gay activist" in the conservative administration.[118]

The fraying of the state's AIDS alliance further diverted energy and resources that might otherwise have been directed at stemming the epidemic in black communities. In the late 1980s, to create a progressive AIDS infrastructure in a conservative state, David Jolly had developed an alliance of likeminded colleagues who had helped ensure the survival of AIDS exceptionalism in North Carolina.[119] Among these were Ron Levine (the state health director), Rebecca Meriwether (the state communicable disease director), and Chris Hoke (the state legal affairs chief).[120] Jolly also collaborated with members of North Carolina's AIDS task force, including Trish Bartlett, Sandy Hendrickson, and Wendee Wechsberg, as well as AIDS lobbyist David Jones, on state policy. Other staff—a special assistant in the Health Department, a hiring professional in Human Resources, an administrator in grants and contracts—also greased the wheels in an otherwise intransigent bureaucracy. These people and many more worked, often unheralded, to ensure that North Carolina had relatively progressive AIDS policies.

Perhaps the most important example of this group's collaborative work came in 1989, when the state passed an antidiscrimination measure to protect people with AIDS. In 1988, the state's AIDS task force had reported that many people with AIDS could still lose their jobs, housing, or insurance because of the disease. Such social or economic repercussions had public health implications, the task force argued, because "many people at risk [of HIV infection] will not come forward" for testing and care if those strictures remained in place.[121] Gay men in particular were concerned because North Carolina's record of anti-gay hate crimes, often connected to AIDS-related fear—was the worst in the nation.[122] Among the task force's thirty-seven recommendations (which included $6.5 million for foster care, drug therapy, health insurance, and affordable housing for those with AIDS) was a demand that the legislature ban AIDS discrimination.[123]

An unusual political window had opened. AIDS activists and state employees had been pushing for antidiscrimination rules for two years, but by 1989 even the governor, various legislative committees, and medical associations supported them.[124] "Politically, there's a great deal of pressure to move . . .," AIDS lobbyist David Jones told reporters. "Two years from now, that impetus is not going to be there."[125] Consequently, legislators in both state houses began floating various legislation.[126] The push was not without controversy, of course. Some Republicans and conservative Democrats considered the effort a "thinly disguised gay-rights bill" that attacked free enterprise and confused state priorities. Some activist AIDS groups deemed the main bill too conservative because it made HIV a reportable condition and left some loopholes open for discrimination.[127] But by 1989, rates of new infection in North Carolina threatened to surpass national averages, and health officials were calling for expanded surveillance strategies to stem the epidemic. Even those who feared that antidiscrimination legislation was a pretext for gay rights could understand the public health benefits the measure provided, while David Jones convinced his allies in the AIDS community that the measure, while imperfect, was their best option.[128] In the fall of 1989, AIDS activists and public health workers had obtained their antidiscrimination bill.

Achieving the antidiscrimination bill may have been the last major victory for Jolly's AIDS exceptionalist alliance, however. Previously, Jolly and his allies had collaborated because they saw AIDS as a common and compelling enemy and because they agreed—for practical or ideological reasons—on the best strategies to address it. By the late 1980s, however, new AIDS therapies, more AIDS workers, and reduced AIDS stigma created tensions within the alliance as gay activists maintained their stand on anonymous testing and noncoercive interventions while public health professionals began exploring more traditional health strategies.[129]

David Jolly had always been able to count on Ron Levine and Rebecca Meriwether to resolve the tensions between public health professionals and gay activists, but by 1989 several forces made this impossible.[130] By this time, half of the states in the country had adopted name-based reporting and contact tracing for HIV, policies buttressed to varying degrees by the CDC and the American Medical Association (AMA).[131] At the same time in North Carolina, conservative health leaders in several counties began voicing their opposition to the state's anonymous-testing policy and received support from the North Carolina Medical Society and the North Carolina Hospital Association.[132] With new reports indicating the drug AZT appeared to delay the onset of AIDS for asymptomatic people, many health professionals began to feel the public health benefits associated with name-based reporting and contact tracing now outweighed the privacy risks involved.[133]

Consequently, many health professionals had supported a provision in the antidiscrimination bill that made HIV reportable, opening a key fissure in the AIDS exceptionalist alliance. Few AIDS activists wanted to implement named-based reporting, and few AIDS clinicians—like John Bartlett at Duke, Charles van der Horst at UNC, and Colin Page in Wake County—wanted to report the names of their clients. But AIDS activists recognized the anti-discrimination bill was the best chance they had to protect people from losing services, employment, or accommodations.[134] Activists chose to back the bill and then worked to convince the Health Services Commission to follow what some other states had done and make HIV reportable in North Carolina by code, rather than by name.[135] The governor and lieutenant governor, however, demanded that the commission outlaw anonymous testing altogether.[136] State health director Ron Levine, caught between these two communities, offered a compromise that would largely stop anonymous testing in the state but would keep fifteen anonymous-testing sites open in various locations so clients could opt for local, confidential testing or regional, anonymous testing if they chose to do so.[137] The Health Services Commission opted for its own compromise, which was to leave anonymous testing sites in every county but mandating that private practitioners report cases. Few were completely satisfied with this resolution, and the Republican administration pledged to take the anonymous-testing debate to the legislature.[138] For their part, AIDS activists no longer knew if they could count on the support of Ron Levine in their exceptionalist alliance. Moreover, the conflict over testing and privacy promised to divert attention away from other issues related to North Carolina's AIDS epidemic.

In the wake of this political skirmish, David Jolly's job grew increasingly uncertain. Administration officials considered him an activist more than a health worker, and Health Department officials loathed his frequent conflicts with more traditionalist disease intervention specialists.[139] On one occasion, Jolly told a group of trainees that "the [health] department was dragging its ass" while a reporter was in the room.[140] The administration was furious when Jolly's remarks hit the front page the next morning. "That hurt me," Jolly acknowledged.[141] Thereafter, the department considered Jolly "a wild card who wasn't always in control of his mouth and someone who wasn't going to tow a party line."[142] Jolly hurt his reputation further when he got into a yelling match with the secretary of Health and Human Services. "I wasn't very politic," Jolly remembered. "And there were people in the room who were just appalled that I did what I did. And probably thought I should have been fired on the spot. But I lost a lot of credibility and so I didn't get invited to a lot of meetings after that."[143] While Rebecca Meriwether kept him from getting fired, Jolly said, "there were certain people who did not want me in the room when major decisions were being made."[144] By 1990, department officials began excluding Jolly from major decisions, and he was passed over for promotion when the department reorganized.[145]

This exclusion proved significant, because it was during Jolly's marginalization that state health leaders chose to abandon the state's anonymous testing program. North Carolina's anonymous HIV testing policy owed its existence and survival to Ron Levine and Rebecca Meriwether, but by 1990 they had changed their views on it.[146] With new therapies available, new protections in place, and new reporting guidelines to implement, Levine and Meriwether had become convinced anonymous testing was no longer necessary. "With these additional [discrimination] protections in place and with new opportunities for medical care," Ron Levine explained to reporters, "we feel the ability to work with patients will be enhanced by knowing who they are."[147] Abandoning anonymous testing would play an important public health role, added Meriwether: "As HIV moves out of the traditional risk groups of homosexuals and intravenous drug users, more of the partners we notify have not acknowledged the risk to themselves. As a result, partner identification becomes a more and more important tool for us to break through that denial of risk so they can begin learning how to protect themselves."[148] Having reached these conclusions, in November 1990 Levine and Meriwether asked the State Health Commission to reduce the number of anonymous-testing sites in 1991 and eliminate them by 1994.[149] During the transitional years between 1991 and 1994, North Carolina would join sixteen other states in offering both anonymous and name-based (or confidential) testing facilities.[150] Many felt this move came out of pressure from the Republican administration, but Levine always maintained that the push "came from the staff: the scientists, the doctors, and the epidemiologists. . . . The staff said this is the right thing to do; they wanted it."[151]

The decision sparked strong opposition from some quarters. Hundreds of people showed up to oppose this policy change at six different state hearings held in early 1991.[152] "There's no way I'm going to tell them my real name and my real address," argued one gay man from Raleigh. " . . . this is a private, intimate thing."[153] "There are many people who I know that would never be tested if it weren't anonymous," added a Charlotte man. The parent of a child with AIDS concluded, "We can not assume the enactment of a law is automatically going to provide confidentiality for those . . . who are HIV infected."[154] AIDS activists were particularly vocal. "They say they need this so they can track these people better and have partner notification," argued a Greensboro activist, "but if people aren't coming in to be tested, then there won't be anyone to notify."[155] "Unless we allow people to be tested anonymously," contended another, "we will see people flock to blood drives to get that same information."[156] "If we are doing such a bang-up job with confidential testing, mandatory contact tracing, and mandatory treatment," asked Wilmington activist Leo Teachout, "[why is] syphilis . . . at an all-time high in North Carolina?"[157] Health workers echoed these complaints. "People are afraid, even with anonymous testing," noted one. "Their fear of disclosure and discrimination is a deterrent to their seeking treatment."[158] "Many people have not been tested before because of the fear of someone knowing," confirmed an HIV counselor from Guilford County. "When we go to confidential testing, that fear is going to be even greater."[159] "I don't know of anyone directly involved in AIDS care that supports this change," concluded an HIV specialist in Winston-Salem.[160] Indeed, in November 1990, the 7,800 member North Carolina Medical Society urged the state to keep some form of anonymous testing.[161]

David Jolly felt deeply betrayed. "I remember meeting at Rebecca Meriwether's house," Jolly later recalled. "I don't know whether they honestly believed it was time or they were reading the political handwriting on the wall and they were given their marching orders. They never said to me. 'Look we have no choice.' They always said to me, 'It's time. The disease is officially destigmatized.'"[162] Jolly felt differently, however: "I just completely disagreed in my heart of hearts. . . . I agreed that there was less stigma in 1990 than there was in 1985, but I just really felt that we needed anonymous testing if we wanted to encourage high-risk gay men to find out their HIV status."[163] Adding insult to injury, Jolly's boss directed him to create the transition plan. "That was the beginning of the end for me," Jolly remembered. Already feeling burned out in his job, insulted by his demotion, and having now been "told to do things [he] just didn't believe in anymore," David Jolly resigned. "It was time," he later concluded. "I left quite happily."[164]

Other sectors supported the policy, however. Mecklenburg County's health director deemed the "phase-out" approach reasonable, and Stanly County's health director considered it a means to reducing AIDS stigma: "We want to provide folks an atmosphere where they can come in and talk to us and feel comfortable doing that."[165] And, while some community and religious leaders backed the policy change, others considered it too moderate. "If it is a good idea four years from now, it is a good idea now," argued Milton D. Quigless Jr., a Raleigh surgeon and co-chairman of a conservative AIDS policy group.[166] Ultimately, Levine and Meriwether's proposal carried the day. At its February 1991 meeting, the North Carolina Health Commission agreed to phase out anonymous testing in eighty-three counties that September, with a total phase-out planned for 1994.[167]

At this point, it is important to understand the extent to which evidence played a role in this debate. AIDS activists frequently claimed that name-based reporting would "drive high-risk individuals underground," but many of these claims were based not on scientifically validated evidence but rather on political negotiation and cultural expectation.[168] When peer-reviewed research did reach the literature in the late 1980s and early 1990s, much of the evidence against name-based reporting was based on opinion surveys of at-risk groups rather than on actual outcomes data.[169] It would not be until the late 1990s that more rigorous studies showed little, if any, abstention from testing due to name-based testing in a state.[170] By this time, however, the deep politicization of AIDS made it very difficult to implement outcomes-based public health strategies related to testing. But even if people had been willing to follow outcomes-based guidelines, the baseline data required did not exist at that time.

Convinced, then, of the correctness of their position, AIDS activists (particularly in gay communities) began devoting a tremendous amount of attention to the defense of anonymous testing. The North Carolina branch of the activist group ACT UP (AIDS Coalition to Unleash Power) demonstrated at the

February commission meeting.[171] They next targeted the legislature and the Department of Public Health.[172] That summer, after Ron Levine announced which counties would retain anonymous testing, AIDS activist and ACRA staff member Lester Lee sued the state on the grounds that the anonymous-testing strategy "was unconstitutional and should be repealed."[173] Durham County was immediately granted an injunction in the case, and the administrative law judge ruled that ACT UP was entitled to a hearing to determine the constitutionality of the state's restricted-testing policy.[174] Eighty-two counties in the state lacked anonymous testing, and a six-year court battle over the issue ensued.

IN ADDITION TO THE VARIOUS structural factors putting African American communities at greater risk for HIV infection and the numerous institutional factors drawing attention away from efforts to address HIV/AIDS in African American communities, important community deficits erected barriers to a vibrant anti-AIDS campaign from within the African American community: generalized homonegativity, middle-class intransigence, a lack of community awareness, religious reluctance or opposition, and historical mistrust of the medical community.

Perhaps the most significant barrier to battling AIDS within black communities, as mentioned above, was the lack of awareness among African Americans about the nature of the problem. As Cullen Gurganus, director of Raleigh's ASA, noted, his group had done a poor job of reaching out to the black community; but when they did, they found that blacks were unaware "about the nature and extent of the illness."[175] "Blacks don't educate," contended one Raleigh AIDS volunteer, "and this will happen to all heterosexuals if they don't educate more . . . more people are going to die."[176] What accounted for this ongoing lack of awareness? Christian Davis-McCoy, an African American AIDS educator in Durham, asserted at the time that "the black community has been overwhelmed and bombarded with other problems . . . [like] teen violence, poverty and discrimination" and that these had slowed their mobilization around AIDS.[177] Compounding this, argued Durham health activist John Mickle, "AIDS is perceived as a gay and a white problem" in black communities, which limited community engagement on the issue.[178]

Even when African Americans were aware of the growing impact of AIDS in some black communities, they did not act immediately. The Kaiser Foundation's Mark Smith argued that while gay communities from top to bottom had "been interested in and involved with AIDS," the epidemic had "hit a segment of the black population about which the official leadership is at best ambivalent. They [did not] have an interest in presenting these people as representative of the problems of their community."[179] Christina Gibbie Harris, prevention program manager for North Carolina's Department of Environment, Health and Natural Resources, concurred: "[It was] not as easy for the black community to organize as for the gay community. There's not that base."[180] Mandy Carter, a black lesbian activist connected to LGHP, maintained that the "stigma associated with AIDS in the black community [was] even stronger than among whites . . . [because of] a number of factors: a fear of revealing weakness, fear of further alienation from society, and most importantly, the silence of the black churches, . . . [who] are loathe to acknowledge the presence of 'immoral' behavior in their community."[181] "In the white community, the more income you have, the less likely you are to be discriminating against gay people," AIDS educator Garry Lipscomb argued.

> In the black community, it is quite the opposite. So folks who are lower income are much more accepting of the gay community than middle class folks. . . . In the black community, it is much more likely that if I am poor, I am going to say, "you have something, go right ahead, I don't have a problem with that." Whereas the middle-class community is more like, "I have to set an example and I have to be much more above this fray. I can't be involved with all that." Then there is the religious community, of course. . . . So if you are in the church, you definitely aren't going to be accepting, and if you are in the middle-class community you are not going to be accepting. That's the big power base for the majority of the black community, the political power base. So . . . yes, there were a lot of people getting infected, but people were trying real hard to ignore it—in the black community.[182]

As Lipscomb's comments suggest, many considered black churches key to the response (or lack thereof) of black communities to HIV/AIDS. Christian Davis-McCoy lamented that while "the black church is in a position of great responsibility [and] it has traditionally been the tool for change . . . they haven't taken the lead with this."[183] "With black churches particularly there was a real issue whether they should leave it alone or whether they should just condemn the whole thing," Howard Fitts remembered.

> Some black churches designated people in the church to . . . have some responsibility. And . . . there were some churches, even at that time, that employed people to help them or to do something in terms

of AIDS education. But most of them [said], "No." . . . [What] we did was to hold workshops with ministers . . . about what their approach could be for AIDS education . . . to help them make the decision that it was all right for them to be concerned about AIDS education and what happened to people with AIDS. You see . . . this was seen as a curse by many people. God's [curse against] homosexuality! . . . But we found pretty good acceptance among ministers if you could get to them individually, and then get them in groups where other ministers showed evidence of being progressive about things. It was less difficult for them then.[184]

According to Louise Alston, however, "less difficult" did not mean easy. "I had a hard time getting into . . . the churches," Alston remembered. "The church, I felt, was the best place to talk about HIV. Where else would you find so many black people on a Sunday morning but in the church? But the pastors didn't want to talk about it. . . . We had one or two pastors here in Durham would talk about it from the pulpit. The rest of them, 'No Sir! Don't want to talk about it, Sister Louise!' . . . [These pastors] weren't educated themselves and . . . they thought that they didn't have anyone in their church [who had AIDS]. That didn't need to be talked about."[185] Indeed, as professor of black religion C. Eric Lincoln explained in 1989, "The church does not necessarily see itself as in the business of rescuing people who go outside its teaching."[186]

Alston felt passionately that churches needed to talk about AIDS. If pastors refused to address it, Alston knew how she could get church people to listen:

[So] I said, "Ok, no problem." Because I know who . . . runs the church: them old sisters, the missioners. . . . So if they weren't going to let me in the front door, I was going to go through the back door. I went through the back door and talked to them old sisters and see what I found when I did that, there was a whole lot of old people in the church that . . . had kids, they had family members who had been diagnosed or use drugs. . . . So when they heard my story and by that time I had gotten my mama to done go with me so mama is telling them how she felt when her son was diagnosed and how she feels now with him died. They listened. They said, "Okay sister. Come on in. We're gonna let you talk." And that's how I got in the church. . . . And they want to hear because either their grandchild or one of their children is in that predicament, and they want to know what to do. "What can I do? I'm tired of it being a secret. I don't know how to help my child. I don't know what to do for my child. I don't know how to talk to my other grandchildren." . . . I have gone and spoke a lot of times on women's day. Cause they would get you in there on some kind of program.[187]

Other community factors came into play. Homophobia was one factor. "People who are infected because of drugs are reluctant to come forward because they don't want to be branded as gay," Christian Davis-McCoy explained to reporters.[188] Fears related to AIDS treatment was another: "Many of the people we deal with don't know that HIV exists in their families. Of those families in which we know HIV exists, many do not want their children tested. Many who know their children are HIV-positive do not want them treated," noted Chris Weedy, a social worker with Duke's Pediatric Infectious Disease Department.[189] Historic suspicions about the mainstream health system also prevailed. Charles van der Horst, at UNC's AIDS clinic, found he frequently had to assure his patients "that they are receiving effective care and are not being used as guinea pigs."[190] Some African Americans feared HIV itself was a conspiracy against African Americans. According to Garry Lipscomb,

> Most people thought that AIDS was an experiment gone bad. The whole conspiracy thing was real big in the African American community. . . . "Someone created this, the CIA, the FBI somebody did that. And they were trying to get rid of us." . . . I mean they thought something was going on here because there are way too many black people getting this. Everybody was still saying this was a gay disease, but at that point, it was not just the black gay men who were getting it. Yes, there were a lot, but people were very clear that it wasn't just gay people in the black community. There were women getting it. The whole sickle cell community was really up in arms with that because a lot of folks were getting infected through blood transfusions.[191]

On top of all of these challenges, AIDS workers had a very difficult time reaching African Americans at risk for HIV-transmission, such as drug users. "In our clinic, we used to see a lot of sexually transmitted diseases among the gay community. Now we see almost none," Erving Hoffman, clinical coordinator for the Durham County Health Department, told reporters in early 1991. In the previous year, 75 percent of new infections occurred among African Americans, and "most of these were IV drug users or partners of IV drug users."[192] Indeed, throughout the state in the early 1990s, African Americans constituted between 66 and 76 percent of newly reported cases.[193] The "lifestyle changes and preventive measures" that were working for many white gay communities had not translated to these other groups.[194] "It's harder to convince these people to change their habits," Christian Davis-McCoy commented. "They're sick and they're addicted."[195]

Outreach to minority women also proved difficult. In the early 1990s, about 15 percent of North Carolinians with AIDS were women, though the number varied by region. Black women accounted for more than 80 percent of these cases.[196] "In terms of our client population, probably about a third are women right now," Jacquelyn Clymore, head of the AIDS Services Agency for Wake County, explained to reporters.[197] Many of the care and prevention strategies aimed at white gay men proved incompatible with the needs of black women at risk for HIV. Few prevention resources were available to them: There are no prevention efforts [aimed at women] right now," the LGHP's Stan Holt admitted to reporters in 1992. "They're not targeting women."[198] Most men in gay relationships had equal negotiating power in terms of AIDS prevention, whereas many women in heterosexual relationships did not: many found themselves vulnerable to the virus because they depended financially on their partner or were trapped in abusive relationships where they lacked the power to insist on monogamy or condom use.

Few AIDS programs were prepared to address the complex set of care needs many of these women had. By the time most infected women sought medical treatment, they were very sick because they had initially been misdiagnosed, largely because they failed to fit the profile of someone at risk for HIV. Many were single mothers who struggled just to find babysitters so they could attend their doctor's visits, much less find someone willing to care for their children after they died. Several small-scale programs did begin in the early 1990s, however: the Woman's Center of Raleigh started a support group for women with AIDS in 1991, the AIDS Services Agency of Wake County launched one in 1992, and both Charlotte Hospice and MAP established childcare programs so women with AIDS could make time to see their doctors.[199] The fact remained, however, that North Carolina lacked any substantive strategy to reach women at risk for or living with HIV. "I called the AIDS Hotline and I knew I was talking to someone gay," a woman with HIV named Pearl told an interviewer. "I asked to talk to a woman, preferably a minority woman, and he said, 'We just answer the phone randomly.' We definitely do need support groups for women. They're rare."[200]

AIDS organizations also did a poor job reaching black MSM. At the AIDS Clearinghouse, Howard Fitts hoped Louise Alston could rectify the group's historic inability to reach black gays when she joined the staff, but Alston left gay outreach to others ("I did not do any education with gay men," Alston recalled.)[201] In 1991, even Garry Lipscomb—the black MSM working with the LGHP—found he had limited access to high-risk, closeted, black MSM. Desperate, Lipscomb began going anywhere he thought high-risk men might be. "The place where I started doing a lot of outreach at that point was going to the adult bookstores and the street hangouts," Lipscomb remembered.[202]

After a decade, despite a newfound urgency about prevention, diagnosis, and treatment across the state, the HIV epidemic continued spreading feverishly through North Carolina's African American communities. People like Garry Lipscomb began looking for new and more effective strategies to stem the tide.

Ironically, as Lipscomb began working to craft new strategies to reach African Americans at risk for HIV, Howard Fitts's time as an AIDS educator came to an end. "We were funded for, like, three years," Dr. Fitts recalled. "After [that] we were not funded. . . . The division of health services discontinued funding us; . . . we phased out then."[203] Louise Alston continued doing some individual volunteering with various AIDS groups, but eventually poor health halted her activism.[204] Howard Fitts continued working with Durham's AIDS Community Residence Association and, a few years after he joined the board, ACRA opened an apartment building in a predominantly black part of Durham that they named the Fitts-Powell Apartments in his honor. "They claimed that they put my name on the apartment because of the work I'd done in health and AIDS," Fitts recalled. "But I said . . . that they put my name there because they thought they might get better community acceptance."[205]

The brief duration of Fitts's AIDS Clearinghouse epitomized the limited effectiveness of African American AIDS organizations. Underresourced in a growing epidemic, many black AIDS organizations lacked the ability to establish a sustained presence. Turnover of AIDS efforts remained high, and the specific task of educating blacks about AIDS would then pass to other motivated individuals.

CHAPTER 5

THE FUTURE OF A FUTURELESS FUTURE
AIDS and the Problem of Poverty in North Carolina

B arbara's life had already been hard.[1] The single twenty-something already had three children and was living in a housing project near uptown Charlotte when she learned she was pregnant yet again. Over the course of her pregnancy, she came to learn two things: she was having a girl, and she had HIV. The diagnosis left her depressed and unable to sleep. When she told her family, they ostracized her and her new baby, worried that Barbara or the baby might somehow bleed and expose them to infection. Their reaction drove Barbara to isolate herself. "I was afraid of dying and needing other people and them not being there," she explained. The isolation only exacerbated her sense of guilt and sadness, however. "You definitely feel some guilt," Barbara told a reporter. "The biggest thing I face, is not knowing how long I'll live. That's what I worry about and I cry about. I say, 'Lord, let me live until my baby is 18 and I'll do whatever you want.'" For Barbara, AIDS carried profound long-term implications for her and her children.

While activists and politicians debated the most appropriate testing policies for the state, and AIDS organizations struggled to raise awareness in at-risk communities, people like Barbara struggled to navigate the complexities of life with AIDS. "With gay men, AIDS is the predominant problem," Barbara Rein, director of the Metrolina AIDS Project (MAP), explained to reporters in the early 1990s. "For many of these women, HIV is one of a list of very pressing problems that can turn a family upside down." "From a social standpoint, it's as if we have two different epidemics," added Dr. Jim Horton, an infectious disease specialist at Carolinas Medical Center in Charlotte. "One [group] consists of mostly men who will come in with a computer printout of what medications they want to take. But these women frequently have children. . . . This is a social disaster as far as the needs of these kids." "They see their children as being more important than themselves and they're real concerned about what's going to happen to them," concluded Renee Wallace, MAP's case manager for women. For these women, the debates over testing policy seemed worlds away, and concerns about the effectiveness of outreach efforts appeared beside the point. Now diagnosed, women like Barbara labored to fit their new medical problems into an already profound burden of disease and dysfunction. As they looked increasingly to the state's health and social services sector, what they found was a system insufficiently equipped to handle their long-term concerns. Outreach ineffectiveness and secondary debates about testing policy were allowing the epidemic to settle deeper into North Carolina's sociosexual networks. In some communities, the epidemic was becoming endemic, and AIDS workers in the state were falling further behind in their battle against the disease.

FOR PEOPLE LIKE BARBARA, the voluntary surveillance system proved an insufficient mechanism because it relied so heavily on community awareness of risk. In many cases such awareness did not exist. Take prisons; in 1991, a report in the *North Carolina Medical Journal* showed that the voluntary testing regime in North Carolina prisons had uncovered only seventy-two cases of HIV among inmates since the start of the epidemic. Throughout the latter half of the 1980s, AIDS activists had successfully fought to prevent state officials from mandating HIV testing for new and existing prisoners. But in 1989, as noted in chapter 4, AIDS activists worked with a diverse coalition of actors to secure a bill protecting people from AIDS-related discrimination.[2] Although some critics considered the measure a thinly disguised gay-rights bill that attacked free enterprise and confused state priorities, the bill actually made HIV a reportable condition.[3] Policymakers followed up on this bill by initiating an HIV testing program in prisons for all new inmates beginning in 1990. In the first six months of the new program, prison officials uncovered eight times as many cases of HIV/AIDS as they had in the previous five years.[4] The communities most likely to become incarcerated in North Carolina — minorities with some connection to petty crime and the drug trade — had not come to see themselves as high risk for HIV infection, so most of these inmates were learning of their HIV exposure for the first time. What was true of prisoners was true of the larger population. Other studies confirmed that up to 94 percent of infected individuals in North Carolina were unaware they had been exposed to HIV.[5]

Evidence further suggested that the anonymous testing and contact tracing system itself was playing a role in this breakdown of awareness. In 1992, a study published in the *New England Journal of Medicine* indicated that in North Carolina, patient-referred partner notification proved far less effective than provider-based partner notification. Almost 50 percent of those tested never returned for counseling. Among those who did return and participated in contact tracing, those working through providers reached approximately 50 percent of their sexual partners, while those opting for anonymous, voluntary contact reached only 7 percent of their partners.[6] "In this trial," concluded the research team, "leaving the notification of partners up to the subjects (patient referral) was quite ineffective, despite the North Carolina law requiring that partners be notified. Partner notification by public health counselors (provider referral) was significantly more effective."[7]

It is not surprising that doctors felt ambivalent about North Carolina's anonymous testing and reporting system. Debates about the policies played out in the pages of the *North Carolina Medical Journal* on at least two occasions in the early 1990s.[8] Some doctors threw their support behind the North Carolina branch of ACT UP, which called for anonymous testing, while others, who opposed it, spearheaded a conservative AIDS policy group known as Americans for a Sound AIDS Policy.[9] Officially, the North Carolina Medical Society backed the American Medical Association's support of anonymous testing, but in November 1990 they called for laws allowing doctors to test patients for HIV without informed consent.[10] Moreover, polls indicated that 65 percent of North Carolina physicians wanted the right to test patients without their consent, and 87 percent endorsed named reporting of those with positive HIV tests.[11]

Concerns about confidential testing became even more acute in the early and mid-1990s with the emergence of new HIV therapies. Particularly important in this regard was the discovery of drugs that radically reduced mother-to-child transmission. Researchers had known for some time that mothers infected with HIV could transmit the virus to their offspring in utero, perinatally, and through breast milk. By the early 1990s, a growing number of women and their children were becoming infected with HIV in North Carolina (six cases in 1989 and twenty-two cases in 1992) and elsewhere.[12] In North Carolina, surveillance restrictions and gaps in prenatal care kept obstetricians from identifying and monitoring HIV-infected women, however. In 1992 and 1993 doctors were able to identify and test only 60 percent of HIV-exposed children.[13] These surveillance gaps had been acceptable because, other than performing an abortion, clinicians could do nothing to prevent perinatal transmission.[14]

In the early 1990s, however, studies indicated that azidothymidine (AZT or zidovudine) might actually reduce mother-to-child-transmission. AZT had been developed by Burroughs Wellcome in North Carolina, and since September 1986, Duke researchers had been testing the drug's effectiveness in children.[15] By 1992, several studies suggested that antiviral therapy could block the perinatal transmission of HIV, and a large, multicenter study published in 1994 showed that, when compared to placebo, zidovudine cut the incidence of perinatal transmission from 25.5 percent to 8.3 percent.[16]

Duke and UNC researchers immediately implemented zidovudine therapy across the state. Aided by support from the state's Health Department, clinicians identified and tested 90 percent of HIV-exposed mothers in 1994; by year's end, 75 percent of these women were taking zidovudine.[17] The results were dramatic: perinatal transmission rates in the state dropped from 21 percent in 1993 to 8.5 percent in 1994. While some of this drop appears to have occurred naturally (only 18.9 percent of those not receiving zidovudine transmitted the virus in 1994), zidovudine made up the largest factor in the decline (only 5.7 percent of HIV-exposed infants were infected after they received zidovudine).[18] North Carolina legislators seized on these results and immediately crafted a law obligating physicians to recommend HIV testing to all pregnant women.[19] While these changes resulted in more aggressive outreach to high-risk pregnant women, that population remained small and many others at risk for HIV infection still remained unaware of their risk.

The policy emphases in place became particularly important at this stage because, at both the state and federal levels, the political environment took a decidedly conservative turn. In North Carolina, cultural conservatives were able to consolidate power within the Republican Party by the early 1990s, and, in 1994 they won control of the state legislature. It was the first time since the Civil War that Republicans had held such power in North Carolina.[20] Since the Democrat-led legislature had only implemented five of the thirty-seven AIDS policy recommendations made by the 1989 state AIDS task force, AIDS activists expected even less support for their efforts as the Republicans took power.[21]

On one level, AIDS activists had reason for concern. Conservatives strongly supported efforts to expand named HIV testing and they worked adamantly to curtail comprehensive sex education in the public schools. In 1995, conservative legislators floated several bills to these ends.[22] Central to conservative efforts was House Bill 834, the so-called teach abstinence until marriage bill, which called for "parental review of and . . . certain restrictions on any instruction on sexually transmitted diseases or out-of-wedlock pregnancy."[23] As early as 1987, social conservatives had tried to pass similar bills, but had lacked the votes. In 1995, however, they were able to guide the bill through to passage. More liberal legislators tried to weaken the bill, which mandated a statewide "abstinence-only until marriage" curriculum and set a high bar for local communities hoping to opt out, but most of the bill's original provisions stayed intact and the provision passed.[24] AIDS educators and gay activists believed the bill, albeit watered down from its initial form, still gutted the state's existing sex education curricula and replaced it with, as one activists put it, "fear-based misinformation about sexuality and health care."[25]

It is important not to overinterpret the impact of these political changes on North Carolina's AIDS policies, however. First, the ascendancy of social conservatives failed to translate into the feared rollback of promising AIDS policies. Many of the policies had already been normalized within the AIDS policy infrastructure. Durham and Mecklenburg Counties, for example, had come to rely on outreach strategies they had originally opposed, such as the use of public money for the dissemination of safer sex materials (including the promotion and distribution of free condoms) and clean needle promotion (whether through bleach kit programs or educational brochures).[26] Likewise, communities across the state had started to embrace low-cost AIDS housing; by 1995, over 120 units for people with AIDS had been established across the state (thirty rooms in various homes, fifty-seven federally funded apartments, and over thirty "temporary shelters").[27] The state government also continued efforts pioneered by David Jolly and Rebecca Meriwether to partner with community-based organizations in the effort against AIDS.[28]

Second, and perhaps more important, it is not clear whether changes in the political landscape fundamentally changed North Carolina's approach to HIV. I have suggested that, in North Carolina, AIDS activists and policymakers prioritized the values of liberty, privacy, and autonomy in their fight against AIDS. The fight over anonymous testing was perhaps the most eloquent embodiment of this perspective, but the preeminence of individual concerns lay at the heart of AIDS exceptionalist policies. Indeed, supporters argued that safeguarding individual concerns was the most effective way to meet collective needs. Critics, however, complained that the preeminence of individual concerns trumped collective concerns. Social conservatives and public health traditionalists often positioned themselves as providing an alternative approach, calling for more interventions that placed the public good above concerns about individual liberties. Proponents of this approach usually argued that the nature of AIDS compelled public health officials to employ coercive tactics—like mandatory testing, named reporting, and named contact tracing—to safeguard public health.

Both groups, however, were largely debating the best ways to address individual behavior change. Gay activists and public health progressives felt that voluntary measures would best bring those at risk into the health system;

conservatives and public health traditionalists believed more coercive measures were necessary. Activists focused on protecting individuals from a discriminatory society in order to promote health; conservatives concentrated on protecting society from diseased, immoral, or irresponsible people. In North Carolina, neither activists nor conservatives devoted much attention to the sociostructural factors that put various groups at risk for ill health in general and AIDS in particular. Individuals can assure their health and protection—from AIDS and other diseases—only in communities that provide meaningful assurance and protections of health. Aligned as they were to the political left, AIDS activists were more ideologically drawn to addressing these social determinants of health than their conservative counterparts; indeed, the efforts around anonymous testing and contact tracing were arguably meant to address some of the sociostructural issues faced by men who have sex with men (MSM). The role discrimination played in the epidemic was difficult to ascertain: most activists argued it impeded or delayed MSM's willingness to access the health system for care and prevention, but many also felt stigma and discrimination actually put MSM at greater risk of HIV acquisition because men might keep their sexual orientation or infection status secret, increasing the odds that risky behavior would occur. Regardless, the problem of discrimination against homosexuals and people with HIV was one of activists' main concerns, often overshadowing many other social factors that raised HIV risks. The problem was, it was by no means clear that one could adequately address these other social determinants if one was already committed to the primacy of individual privacy and noncoercive interventions.

The issue of HIV in prisons provides an example. AIDS activists had long fought against mandatory HIV testing of inmates because it violated their right to privacy, while conservatives and public health traditionalists called for it. Under the AIDS exceptionalist regime, corrections officials and health workers had only identified infected inmates late in their disease progression. After corrections officials and conservative politicians secured mandatory HIV testing of all new inmates, it became clear that hundreds of inmates had passed through prisons with asymptomatic infections. In the years that followed, those on both the political left and right supported increased funding for HIV treatment and surveillance in prisons. This was not an insignificant move. Investing in HIV treatment in prisons provided inmates with access to care they might not otherwise have received outside the corrections system. But as discussed in the previous chapter, prisons posed a double dilemma for the HIV epidemic: they increased the spread of HIV because of the risks to which they exposed inmates and inmate communities, and they furthered racial HIV disparities because blacks were overrepresented in North Carolina prisons. One feasible means to address HIV in prisons might have been to propose alternate sentencing guidelines for nonviolent drug offenders so that those inmates and their communities would be safe from HIV exposure. Or North Carolina might have decriminalized (though not legalized) drugs, shifting budgetary outlays from corrections to substance abuse therapy. These kinds of measures were not a priority for AIDS activists, and they proved incompatible with many conservatives' more traditional "tough on crime" stance.

AIDS activists, who might have been politically predisposed to address the social determinants of health, gave political primacy to issues of individual privacy, which prevented them from addressing these larger issues. For their part, conservatives were politically indisposed to address the social determinants of health, but they, too, gave political primacy to certain individualist values. And so, in North Carolina, responsibility for HIV policies shifted from those who could have addressed the social determinants of health through the legislature but failed to do so to those who had little interest in addressing the social determinants of health at all.

THE RISE OF SOCIAL CONSERVATIVES in North Carolina's political infrastructure did not mean that HIV/AIDS efforts became starved of resources. The flood of federal and state funds, best embodied by the Ryan White CARE Act, brought a host of mainstream health providers into North Carolina's AIDS funding stream. Beginning in 1991, the Ryan White CARE Act began pumping almost $1 million into North Carolina, $684,000 of which the state designated for the nine HIV care consortia that covered 80 percent of the state.[29] By 1994, there were fifteen consortia, and each channeled funds to groups as diverse as community hospitals, local United Way groups, church committees, and housing organizations.[30] By 1996, as many as thirty different AIDS Service Organizations existed in North Carolina.[31] Many of these received funding through state or local agencies.

Rather than providing an impetus to expand the focus on social determinants of health, this influx of money changed the relationships that AIDS organizations had with one another and it tempered and normalized AIDS care and control strategies by integrating them more easily into the preexisting health structure. The relationship between AIDS group changed because the flood of money introduced unprecedented competition between groups for the limited amount of local dollars available. Groups like the Lesbian and

Gay Health Project (LGHP), who had experienced relatively easy access to federal funds during David Jolly's tenure, now found themselves competing with numerous other groups for the same pool of funds. "I am absolutely sick of all this competition," LGHP director Stan Holt complained to his board in 1993, after the North Carolina Health Department opened AIDS grant programs "to all community-based organizations."[32] Many groups, including the LGHP, struggled just to survive. And some groups, like the AIDS Clearinghouse, were forced to close their doors. Groups like the LGHP entered into cooperative arrangements with other groups in order to survive. In the LGHP's case, they began in 1992 to talk with the AIDS Services Agency of Wake County, Orange County AIDS workers, and the Triangle AIDS Interfaith Network about collaborating to compete for a larger share of federal funds.[33]

Collaborations entailed several tradeoffs. On one hand, they enabled smaller groups to compete more effectively with larger organizations. They also could potentially increase efficiencies and reduce redundancies. On the other hand, the competitive pressures threatened to homogenize group approaches to AIDS and dilute innovative outreach efforts with more mainstream talk about "service delivery." Groups aligned with county health departments or the United Way were less likely to analyze AIDS through the lens of race, class, or gender.[34] AIDS educators aligned with mainstream non-profit groups or state health offices had less incentive to push back against state "offensiveness" guidelines or to experiment with culturally appropriate outreach language.[35] AIDS organizations looking to foundations and pharmaceutical companies for support found it easier to concentrate on delivering services, and to leave social critique to groups like ACT UP.[36] And while the collaborative competition allowed smaller groups more opportunity to compete, the advantage still tipped toward larger organizations. Unlike small groups, not only did they already have an infrastructure in place to handle a significant influx of funds, but they also were better equipped to address the changing nature of the epidemic by switching from outreach, education, and prevention services to treatment when it became available. In addition, larger organizations were also able to claim some measure of diversity, owing to the demographics of their clientele, regardless of whether the administrative leadership reflected any substantial diversity in perspective or approach.[37]

As AIDS care and prevention services began to mirror North Carolina's larger health service apparatus, they increasingly reflected the weaknesses inherent in North Carolina's delivery system. The burgeoning AIDS funding stream, sent into overdrive with the passage of the Ryan White CARE Act, augmented existing health delivery services or created parallel new ones for numerous communities across the state. In the early 1990s, for example, the Durham County Health Department was able to use federal funds to open an Early Intervention Clinic at the Lincoln Community Health Clinic, the city's primary health provider for low-income Durham residents.[38] The facility wedded HIV care to the larger health system by providing continuity of care for people with HIV in the same location that many of them received their other health services. At the state level, North Carolina began setting aside money so people with AIDS could buy AIDS drugs. Since 1987, the state had used federal funds to provide drugs to low-income and uninsured individuals.[39] In 1993, the number of people needing medication outstripped the funds available, and the state earmarked $200,000 to make up the difference; by 1995, that number had climbed to $450,000.[40] The state also initiated a Housing Opportunities for Persons with AIDS (HOPWA) Predevelopment Loan Program at this time to provide new housing for persons with AIDS. In 1995, they launched a HOPWA Rental Assistance Program that allowed people to remain in their homes or access private housing units when their illness deprived them of an income.[41]

While these funding mechanisms filled gaps or created new services for people with AIDS, they also highlighted the troubling disparities in health care access and outcomes that existed in North Carolina's health care infrastructure. Health disparities occur wherever specific subpopulations bear a significantly disproportionate burden of disease when compared to other subpopulations or the general population.[42] Frequently, these disproportionate burdens fall on members of certain minority groups or socioeconomic strata. Evidence suggests that disparities in health outcomes proliferate in nations with high degrees of economic inequality, but these disparities have been augmented in the United States because of its piecemeal health insurance system.[43] North Carolina already had a variety of problems in this regard. According to the North Carolina Center for Health Statistics, in 1993, the rate of heart disease among black males was 1.4 times higher than that among white males, and the rate of cerebrovascular disease was 3 times as high.[44] In addition, the cervical cancer mortality rate among black women was two and a half times that among white women, and the diabetes incidence rate was three times that for white women.[45] This higher incidence of disease corresponded with lower health care access and utilization. Compared to white women, black women were one-third less likely to receive prenatal care before the fourth month of pregnancy, four and a half times more likely not to have any prenatal care at all, and 11 percent more likely to be diagnosed at a later stage of cervical cancer.[46] Moreover, in the early 1990s, 27 percent of African Americans in North Carolina lived below the federal poverty line; so many black communities in the state bore the double burden of racial and economic health disparities.[47]

In large measure, HIV fit into these preexisting patterns of disease disparity across the state. By early 1993, all but six rural counties were reporting cases of AIDS in the state, prompting the Centers for Disease Control and Prevention to upgrade North Carolina from a "low incidence" to "moderate incidence" state. African Americans continued bearing the brunt of the disease. Sixty-five percent of all new HIV infections occurred among African Americans, and 56 percent of all adult cases affected African Americans, despite the fact that blacks constituted only 22 percent of the state population.[48] With HIV/AIDS, African Americans were again experiencing an excess of disease-specific morbidity and mortality.

The ease with which HIV fell into the preexisting patterns of disease disparity revealed the extent to which sociostructural factors were putting black communities at risk for HIV/AIDS. Health disparities are a downstream phenomenon, that is, they are symptomatic of fundamental problems in the health of populations. As I have already shown, several structural factors, including poverty, violence, drug addiction, community disruption, increased HIV risks in black communities. As North Carolina's epidemic stretched into its second decade, the connection between these factors and the spread of HIV became increasingly clear.

In North Carolina's urban centers, AIDS groups still struggled to get AIDS messages to minority communities effectively. Black MSM proved particularly difficult. Data drawn from North Carolina's major cities between 1990 and 1995 indicated that between 40 and 55 percent of new HIV cases occurred among black MSM.[49] Transmission between black gays constituted between 25 and 35 percent of all infections among African American men during this period.[50] Despite these trends, state health officials reported that "most community-based organizations serving [MSM] have either all or nearly all white staffs, limiting effectiveness among men of color who are at risk," and found that much of the material used for these special populations was of "limited usefulness."[51] Groups like the LGHP, who were so successful in reaching white gay men, never saw similar success in their outreach efforts to black gays. Between 1989 and 1992, African American men constituted 30 to 40 percent of all MSM with HIV in the Triangle, but they never constituted more than 17 percent of the MSM contacted by LGHP.[52]

Obstacles remained even when the LGHP directed attention to black MSM. In 1993, LGHP secured funds and hired Garry Lipscomb to head a minority effort called Black Men United. Lipscomb was a social worker with a long volunteer history with the group. After coming on board, Lipscomb quickly saw how difficult it had been for LGHP to reach black MSM: many did not consider themselves gay (to them, "gay" meant effeminate men dressing like women and adopting receptive sexual roles); few saw themselves at risk for the disease; and most had little contact with the larger gay community (they frequented parks and liquor houses rather than the gay bars they could not afford).[53] Abandoning LGHP's traditional model, Lipscomb targeted certain street corners and park hangouts, where he knew some black MSM would exchange money for sex. "[They] were selling themselves to make money to live," Lipscomb explained, "so they could have a place to live, so they could have food to eat. . . . Those folks were really living hand to mouth; . . . [others] were selling their bodies for drugs."[54] Lipscomb also took condoms and prevention materials to particular gay bookstores that black men frequented for anonymous sex.[55] Additionally, Lipscomb conducted peer education in local liquor houses, which, Lipscomb explained, were homes in black communities where poor people could get "marijuana, cocaine, [some] heroin . . . [and] lottery tickets. Pretty much anything that was illegal that could be sold was being sold. . . . This was their entertainment for the week. They were blowing most of their earnings. . . . They weren't saving for retirement. . . . They weren't going to be having a whole bunch of these evenings for the next couple of weeks."[56] House managers, who saw "their clientele were dying," let Lipscomb discuss safer sex practices with patrons. This frequently proved delicate: "Some people just were not interested. They didn't want to talk about it at all. If I scared off enough people, then the [owner] would say, 'Okay, you got to go.'"[57] Even with a creative black educator finding scores of previously unreached men, outreach efforts to black MSM proved slow and ineffective.

One of Lipscomb's key challenges was to reach young black men engaged in what has been called "exchange sex," "patronage sex," or "transactional sex," that is, individuals who entered sexual relationships with older men not so much for the purpose of survival but rather for increased access to the accoutrements of a higher standard of living: clothes, money, housing, and social circles to which they might not otherwise have access.[58] While these individuals exposed themselves to a higher risk of transmission than someone who lacked such "arrangements," Lipscomb frequently found that the lifestyle incentives made available to these young men in these relationships outweighed any concerns they might have about acquiring a long-latency disease. This group of young men fell so far outside LGHP's prevention model that they proved almost impervious to outreach: few frequented gay bars, many did not identify as gay, most traveled in subterranean social circles, most belonged to asymmetrically structured sexual relationships, and few felt much incentive to "eroticize" condom use to the detriment of their arrangements. These men proved to be some of the most difficult individuals for Lipscomb to reach in Durham.

AS THE EPIDEMIC DUG IN to black urban communities, it also began to spread rapidly through North Carolina's rural minority communities. AIDS had touched almost every county in the state by the early 1990s. Initially, the AIDS cases that surfaced in rural communities consisted of infected people who had returned home from other parts of the country to receive care from their families and to die. These "immigrants" made up almost two-thirds of the first wave of rural AIDS cases.[59] The demographics had changed by the early 1990s, however, as rural health workers began seeing the number of "'home-grown' patients" eclipse the "immigrant" AIDS population.[60] Between 1991 and 1992, AIDS rates in communities with populations lower than 50,000 rose 9.4 percent.[61]

Clinicians in eastern North Carolina were the first to begin chronicling the spread of AIDS into rural communities. In 1991, Richard Rumley, an infectious disease doctor in Greenville, published an article in the journal *AIDS* noting that "there was a striking rise in the number of new AIDS and HIV patients [in rural eastern North Carolina]: cases are doubling approximately every 12 months while the AIDS incidences in New York State reached a plateau in mid-1989 and in North Carolina in early 1990."[62] According to Rumley, AIDS in rural North Carolina had some very specific contours: "The most significant difference between our patient population and the North Carolina and New York State populations is the increased proportion of non-whites in [our] population. [Additionally,] heterosexual transmission is more common than homosexual transmission."[63] The trends Rumley identified only worsened in the years to follow, especially in the rural counties along the I-95 corridor.[64]

Rumley's was something of a unique story. Born in Greensboro and raised in Reidsville, North Carolina, Rumley grew up in a relatively impoverished environment. "My mommy was a nurse; my daddy was a drunk. And basically we had absolutely no money," Rumley explained in an interview in 2010. "My daddy spent more time drunk and in jail then he spent sober."[65]

Along with his troubled family life, Rumley faced other challenges. "[For the] first six years of my life, I was called retarded. . . . Now its called dyslexia, but I was in the 'retarded' class." In that context, Rumley's mother had very low expectations for him. "My mother thought, 'well, you know, shoot, if you can graduate from high school and get a job sweeping floors you'll be doing pretty good,'" Rumley recalled.[66] As it turned out, some of the lawyers and judges in town who frequently dealt with Rumley's father became Rumley's benefactors. He was able to graduate high school, attend college at the University of North Carolina at Chapel Hill, and go on to pursue graduate studies in medicine and immunology.[67] After doing a residency in Mississippi, Rumley ended up in eastern North Carolina at East Carolina University's Brody School of Medicine.

Within a year of arriving in eastern North Carolina, Rumley began seeing AIDS patients. He had seen his first such patients back in Mississippi as early as 1979, though of course they were not called AIDS patients at the time. As a newly minted infectious disease attending physician, these cases fell to him. In part, this was because few other physicians at the hospital wanted to address it. "You know," Rumley recalled, "shit rolls down hill, and I was on the bottom." Additionally, few people thought AIDS would be a problem in eastern North Carolina. "It was something we thought, 'Well, we're in a little rural area. It's not going to be a problem here; it's going to go away,'" Rumley remembered.[68] Finally, Rumley saw the care of vulnerable people to be his calling. Since his time spent with developmentally disabled students in elementary school, Rumley had become something of a "socially conscious monster." "Some of my best friends were people nobody wanted to be around," Rumley explained, "[so] I became a human sanitation engineer . . . someone who fought vehemently for those people who weren't acceptable."[69] This perspective was cemented during his time in Mississippi seeing indigent patients. "I could take those people and admit them to . . . the hospital for three days, and hook them up with social services, and [they] absolutely would turn their life around," said Rumley, " . . . I could really make a difference." So, in the mid-1980s, Rumley became the AIDS doctor in eastern North Carolina. "Since I was kinda one of these people who was sympathetic . . . I was not only at the bottom of the hill, but I was kind of a vacuum for these people in this sort of space."[70]

Unlike what people imagined, however, AIDS in eastern North Carolina proved neither rare nor temporary. "I kept doing more and more and more and more," Rumley explained. "In the late 80s, early 90s, I was burying two or three people a day, twenty-four/seven. . . . . I'm talking about weekends, too. I mean, they were dying."[71] At first, the hospital was uncomfortable with its growing role in AIDS care. "When we were trying to ask for help and assistance," Rumley recalled, "[hospital administrators] said, 'No, we're not going to do that, you'll invite 'em here.'"[72] At the time, Rumley explained, AIDS was highly stigmatized. People in eastern North Carolina, as elsewhere, did not like it and wanted nothing to do with it. The medical center initially discouraged Rumley and his colleagues from applying for grant funding. "The problem with grants is a couple of things," Rumley explained. "One is, usually they are matching grants, and [hospital administrators] didn't want to match it. The other thing is that they didn't want to create a system where [AIDS patients] could easily come here and be taken care of. They didn't want to attract them. They wanted to make it as hard as they could to be here."[73]

The medical center could not ignore the problem for long, however, because the problem was growing in eastern North Carolina, and Bowman Gray Hospital was where AIDS patients all came. "There are 29–30 counties that feed into Pitt County, and so all the AIDS patients in that area came here," Rumley explained. "[So] we kept saying, 'Listen, they're coming here no matter what. If we don't get ready for them, they're just going to clog up our emergency rooms and be found dead in the parking lot. It's going to look bad on you.'"[74] Finally, Rumley and his colleagues were able to browbeat hospital administrators into permitting them to obtain grants.

With a growing number of AIDS cases and limited resources, Rumley's boss went to speak with policymakers in Raleigh about funding. Rumley explained, "My partner at that time, Harry Adams, who was chief of Infectious Diseases . . . went up and spoke to the governor (it was [James] Martin at the time). . . . I wasn't there but [Harry Adams] said, 'The governor says there is no AIDS in eastern North Carolina.' Then we developed this total global saying, that 'there is nothing east of I-95.' It sounds funny, but it's true. . . . [And] that kind of made me say, 'We've gotta let people know there is AIDS here.'"[75] As a result of Adams's meeting with the governor, Rumley determined to document AIDS's presence in eastern North Carolina. The data he gleaned formed the basis for the aforementioned *AIDS* article.

Rumley's study highlighted several of the intersecting factors involved in the spread of HIV into rural minority communities: poverty, drug use, violence, high-risk sexual relationships, and unstable domestic arrangements. From the very beginning, the majority of these patients were black. "I-95 connects to New York City and Miami, and I-95 is an easy way to get from place to place," Rumley explained. "[These people] grew up here, but they went to New York to get a job, . . . didn't get successful, got AIDS, came back home. Some of them sick, some of them not."[76] While Rumley did see some white gay men who had come home to be cared for by their families, their numbers were small, and their doctors frequently referred them to Duke or UNC Chapel Hill. According to Rumley,

> Most of the African Americans [who came back] were drug addicts, although some were bisexual drug addicts, and most of them were really burned out. . . . Those [who were] sick would come right to the hospital. Those not sick would go out and . . . fuck their heads off, and everyone else's, and share needles, etc., and those people basically brought it back. And in a way, 'cause a lot of them that were in the city were streetwise and they were charming, and so the local people were just kinda prey. Not that either one of them were being mean to each other. They were prey."[77]

According to Rumley, poverty proved key to the rural AIDS epidemic.[78] Behind all the pretty cornfields that stood along the highways of eastern North Carolina were rundown houses or trailers where people barely made ends meet. Life was very difficult for many of these impoverished people, a disproportionate number of whom were African American. "Take a common example," Rumley explained in a 1994 article,

> A young man who grows up in poverty, and despised, as "just another drain on the system." Why not sell illegal drugs? Drugs bring ready money, respect from peers, and buy the things you want. The law, jail and violence are just occupational hazards. Besides, they add excitement to a job. Or, take a 14-year-old girl, similar upbringing and surroundings to the young man we discussed. Why put sexual relations off? It is fun. It feels good now and offers a close human relationship. And, what if she happens to get pregnant? We as a society treat pregnant women with goddess status. So immediately she has been elevated from the dung-heap to Princess. Why put pregnancy off? And, when she delivers she has the love and dependence of her child. It is no surprise to me that drugs, violence, prostitution, and recreational sex are commonplace since they offer ready income, immediate escape, pleasure and social elevation. . . . It is no wonder that teenagers and young adults in these hopeless surroundings are forced to look for immediate fulfillment of these needs; even if this search exposes them

to the threat of AIDS, unwanted pregnancy, drug addiction, jail or a violent death to fulfill these needs.[79]

Risky sexual behavior figured prominently in this sociostructural context. Individuals in rural counties engaged in riskier sex than their urban counterparts: fewer used condoms, while more had multiple sex partners, engaged in concurrent sexual arrangements, and acquired sexually transmitted infections.[80] Rumley saw these dynamics firsthand. "When they came back, they brought AIDS and whatnot," he explained. "And then . . . some of them want to live with a person. . . . One of them has AIDS, one of them doesn't. End of the year, both of them have AIDS, and they even have a child that has AIDS. And then they split up . . . and now these two people want to have someone else, so these two people go to two other people. . . . And after a while it's, you know, one person goes to two to four and on and on."[81]

Frequently, these sexual risks and concurrent sexual partnerships overlapped with domestic and sexual violence.[82] Amy, one of the black women profiled in Whetten-Goldstein's *"You're the First One I've Told,"* is a case in point. Rejected by her biological mother for being "too black," Amy was adopted by her aunt and lived most of her childhood feeling more like a servant than a daughter. Amy's father, a violent and abusive alcoholic, worked too infrequently to lift the family out of grinding poverty, and Amy felt little motivation or support to stay in school past the ninth grade. The violence at home was matched by violence in her relationships: around the time Amy dropped out of the tenth grade, her boyfriend and his brothers gang raped her in the woods. Amy ricocheted through several other violent relationships before discovering, in 1991, that she was four months pregnant by her then-boyfriend, who had been incarcerated for the aggravated rape of two girls. During her prenatal care, Amy learned she also had HIV. Devastated by the news of her infection, Amy succumbed to pressure from county health staff and aborted her fetus so she would not have a sick baby to care for.[83] Gina, another woman described in Whetten-Goldstein's book, endured a marriage to an unfaithful and abusive man who infected her with HIV in 1987. Gina did not learn of her infection until 1993, two years after her husband's death, when authorities compelled her to undergo an HIV test after a clinician stuck himself with her nonsterilized needle.[84]

Unstable housing situations in rural areas helped feed these risky sexual behaviors. According to Rumley, "None of [his patients] lived anywhere; everybody "stayed" somewhere. [They would say] 'I "stay" with my sister' [or] 'I "stay" with my brother.' And about every two or three months they would 'stay' somewhere else."[85] This was a problem because if Rumley and his colleagues were ever able to secure Medicaid benefits for these patients, their Medicaid would run out as they moved from place to place and county to county. This transience and instability robbed these individuals of any continuity of care and limited their ability to vote for local policies that might benefit them.

The housing insufficiency of this population highlighted a larger problem for rural residents at risk for HIV/AIDS: they lacked an effective support structure for compliant care. According to Rumley, many of his patients were indigent, "and they had no one willing to take care of them. No one. . . . Hell, the parents didn't even want to come and sit with their children. They would wipe the door handle with a towel before they walked in and after they walked out."[86] Rumley found that his impoverished patients could not "get rides, they can't get medicines, they don't want the medicines ('it makes me sick,' [they'd say]). And . . . they can't keep up assistance because they 'stay' somewhere and they move around. That's kinda the way it is." Beyond this, many of Rumley's rural patients struggled with compliance and fatalism. "Those people that come in the clinic that have AIDS, they're not using protection," Rumley explained. "They're not changing [their behavior], because they say, 'well, you know, if I don't have it, I'm gonna get it, and if I got it, who cares?'"[87]

The isolation associated with rural living only compounded these issues. The counties feeding into Bowman Gray occupied a land mass the size of New Jersey. In the early 1990s, the population totaled only about 1.3 million, so communities were profoundly spread out and lacked any substantive public transportation system.[88] Rural isolation therefore had considerable implications for disease management and disease prevention. Rural HIV patients sought treatment later in the course of their disease, which led to a poorer prognosis, incurring greater costs for their communities and potentially exposing a greater number of other community members to the virus. In addition, many of them considered themselves to be low-risk for HIV transmission precisely because of their rural residence and therefore did not think they needed to worry about condoms or clean needles.

To combat these misapprehensions, Rumley and his colleagues tried to help patients connect to local social services. "We finally got this mapping program . . . to find out who lived where and map the available services around them, so . . . [when] we saw them we could set them up for those things," Rumley explained.[89] Many of Rumley's patients addresses "were nonexistent," so Rumley would have to drive out to their homes, ascertain the latitude and longitude of their houses on a map, and then plug the data into the mapping program "so we could figure out whether or not they . . . would be around someplace that could get them services."[90]

Rumley was not the only one seeing these problems, of course. In Chapel Hill, Charles van der Horst saw numerous rural patients—both black and white—who lived in his region. "The poor patients, they have to travel far," van der Horst told interviewers in 1998. "They don't have transportation, none of them have cars. Most of them do not have phones. I mean everything we take for granted they don't have. . . . They can't afford [certain HIV medications] because they don't have running water."[91] Many rural patients with HIV faced almost insurmountable odds in their effort to manage their disease.

At this stage in the epidemic, the state's health infrastructure was insufficient to meet the needs generated by AIDS in rural communities. Rumley and his team were unable to secure Ryan White funds when they first became available, but they were able to find enough money to launch a local AIDS Service Organization (they called it the Pitt County AIDS Service Organization, or PICASO). In the ensuing years, Rumley and his colleagues supplied data to AIDS advocates in Wake County to form a collaborative venture to secure Ryan White funds. According to Rumley, however, after the Wake group received their Ryan White funds, they limited their services to Wilson County (which includes part of the I-95 corridor and abuts Pitt County). "We felt like they had used our data, which was miserable," Rumley recalled, ". . . and we didn't really get anything out of the Ryan White."[92] Ironically, Rumley was able to make the most of the state's Medicaid rules. "If you were diagnosed with AIDS, then you automatically got Medicaid," Rumley explained. "At the time . . . the definition of AIDS had changed from an opportunistic infection to anybody who had a CD4 count of lower than 250. And a lot of those people weren't sick, and we would get them to apply for Medicaid anyway, 'cause [their illness] met the definition of AIDS."[93] This meant that a lot of Rumley's patients could get assistance for which they might not otherwise have been eligible. Eventually, though, as AIDS therapies improved and the recession of the late 1990s strained local budgets, North Carolina tightened its Medicaid eligibility criteria in this regard.

The general poverty in rural North Carolina, combined with the decentralized nature of medical and social services, meant that the resource constraints already plaguing urban patients became amplified for rural people with HIV/AIDS and their families.[94] Rumley and his team tried to be as flexible as permissable within eligibility rules so they could obtain the most resources for their patients. "[Otherwise] people [weren't] going to be taken care of," Rumley explained.[95] They became experts at navigating the various support systems available to their patients. Rumley and his team were ultimately unwilling to break the rules, however, because they had heard of several AIDS clinics across the country forced to close owing to real or alleged fraud. Recycling AIDS drugs was a case in point. "There were all these people with AIDS [who had] died who had these expensive bottles of drugs, and you . . . you had to throw them away. You couldn't recycle them 'cause it's illegal," Rumley explained. "We didn't do it . . . even though we really wanted to 'cause it would have really helped if we could have done that."[96] Whatever his opinions on the merits of the rules, Rumley feared that his patients would be left with even less support if his team got caught breaking them.

What made such situations even more frustrating for Rumley and his team was that, as urban areas began to see their HIV/AIDS numbers improve, they feared public attention would neglict the escalating problem of AIDS in rural areas.[97] To combat the prospect of neglect, Rumley traveled across eastern North Carolina—visiting schools, churches (both black and white), medical societies, and health education centers—educating health professionals about the problem of rural AIDS and the forces that underlay its spread.[98] His presentation was not particularly sophisticated: "We took the state statistics [and] federal statistics of who lived where, who was in the poverty range, what the racial mix was, and we also took things like reported statistics on gonorrhea and syphilis, TB, and we mapped all those and we laid the maps on top of each other. And they were [a perfect fit]. 'Cause where the Afro-American high densities were is where the poverty was, is where most of our AIDS per capita was coming from, which is also where syphilis, gonorrhea, and TB were."[99] For Rumley, who usually titled his presentation "AIDS as a Disease of Poverty," "it was poverty, it was pure poverty. . . . My talk was basically to show them these maps, and the statistics of the maps told a story. Because when you start going through this thing, start showing one map after the other . . . the root of that was African American. . . . It was race . . . but the race thing—the racism, the bigotry—is just a tool for economics."[100] According to David Jolly, who had left the state AIDS office and met Rumley while working with the North Carolina AIDS Training Network, Rumley's work made it clear that AIDS was "going to devastate African American communities if something [did not] happen . . . not the African American community in general but poor people . . . people [who] didn't have the resources and [who] were being poorly served by the predominantly white gay male HIV/AIDS service organizations."[101]

Rumley's talk met with a variety of responses. Frequently, according to Rumley, "the salt of the earth, nonleaders in the churches, would come up to me and say 'you're so sweet, you're so good' for doing the talk."[102] Church leaders were a different story. Rumley often found black church leaders unwilling to embrace the issue. "A lot of the leaders in black churches did not like [the talk]," Rumley recalled. "Unfortunately, because AIDS is a disease of "bad" people—homosexuals and drug addicts—a lot of the older people in black churches, a lot of the leaders, were not that receptive. . . . I think they felt it was kind of a problem for me to even know about it and to talk to them."[103] One regional leader who was receptive was the pastor of Cornerstone Baptist Church, Sydney Lockes. Lockes, who had also served as a state representative, understood the threat that HIV/AIDS posed to African American communities. "Without him, I don't think we could have gotten anywhere," Rumley concluded. "He helped not only with the grants, [but also] just sometimes by being there" to ensure entrée to black churches.[104]

White churches were even more ambivalent toward people affected by HIV/AIDS. Some people voiced very strong positions: "One of [the comments] I love," Rumley recalled, "was, 'In Cuba, they lock all of these people up. So we ought to have a system like Cuba.'"[105] As was the case at black churches, there were always church members who met Rumley afterward and voiced their support. As often, however, Rumley ran into people in the parking lot "who wanted to speak [in the church] but were afraid to speak in front of the other people because I guess they thought God would get 'em. So they met me in the parking lot and they tried to talk me out of . . . all my beliefs."[106] In an effort to head off some of these confrontations, though also stemming from his personal motivations for his work with AIDS patients, Rumley would include a quotation from Matthew 25:40 in his talks. "That's the one that says, 'when you do it for the least of these, you do it for me,'" Rumley explained. "I wasn't trying to showboat. . . . What I was trying to do was get them to realize that, if God created this virus, . . . God allows people to get it. But the reason that God allows that is not 'cause he hates homos, but because this pain and suffering brings us together."[107]

Rumley met similar resistance at schools, medical societies, and community groups with whom he spoke. Many listeners considered people with AIDS to be bad or lazy. "These are the people that go out and take their social security checks and buy TVs," Rumley remembered many people saying. "And so we shouldn't be helping these people at all." Frequently, Rumley was asked whether he thought "AIDS [was] just taking money away from breast cancer victims."[108] Such resistance in both black and white communities, however, only pushed Rumley to work harder. "You know, it's like missionaries," Rumley explained. "They have this incredible drive to do these crazy things and put themselves in total jeopardy. So that's what I did."[109]

On November 6, 1996, Richard Rumley gave his last talk on AIDS. It had been a busy year: in the previous twelve months, Rumley logged thousands of miles crisscrossing the eastern part of the state delivering 180 versions of his AIDS talk to many different groups. New AIDS therapies were beginning to change AIDS mortality rates, but much of the rest of the AIDS epidemic in North Carolina remained the same, particularly in rural communities. The new infection rate remained steady, existing infections continued being identified far too late in the disease's progression, and the existing infrastructure for care, prevention, treatment, and housing remained inadequate. Rumley had grown discouraged and his audiences had grown jaded. "I went down [to eastern North Carolina] and I did this thing, and the people were lukewarm," he explained. "I tried to throw myself into it . . . [but] I obviously wasn't reaching people anymore."[110] Driving home afterward, Rumley felt God spoke to him. "God told me . . . 'Stop!'" Rumley explained.

> "You don't owe me anything. It's just, what you're doing's worthless. They've learned all the tricks. There's no more tears in the eyes." And I said, "Well you know, nobody's doing this. Nobody believes this. Here I am trying to save the world and the damn world doesn't want to be saved. The rich don't want me to do it, 'cause they like being rich. The poor don't want me to do it, 'cause they're comfortable being poor." Even for the minorities. This was a group that should have been listening. . . . What I think [community leaders] wanted to know at that time was how can we ignore it and still look good? . . . You know, eastern North Carolina is a third world country. Einstein was right: two parallel universes can coexist and not even know the other one exists.[111]

For Rumley, AIDS was just one among many problems ("teenage pregnancies, domestic violence and drugs") that poor communities faced. "These problems can be solved," Rumley wrote in a 1994 article, "when we see that these problems are actually the late terminal symptoms of a 'futureless future.'" Poor children, particularly African Americans, grew up in communities where their existence was despised and they were viewed as "just another mouth to feed."[112] Poor minority communities, whether urban or rural, had little prospect of a substantive or attainable future. Until people from the "two parallel universes" began to see each other, the despair of the "futureless future" remained the most likely possibility for many in poor minority communities.

In this regard, rural AIDS was merely the most pronounced example of the larger problem of health disparities and the social determinants of health in poor minority communities. It also signified the extent to which, up to this stage, HIV care and prevention policy largely overlooked or underaddressed the unique shape of the HIV/AIDS epidemic in minority communities. Black community leaders, white AIDS organizations, state lawmakers, and state health officials all played their various roles in this state of affairs. As a consequence, HIV increasingly became endemic in many black communities in North Carolina.

CHAPTER 6

GET REAL. GET TESTED.

AIDS as a Chronic Disease in the American South

In 1996, over a decade had passed since David Jolly first heard of HIV/AIDS, but there he was, still trying to push North Carolinians to act against the disease. His context had changed considerably. He no longer struggled in isolation: he now served as vice chairman of a blue ribbon panel of health professionals called the North Carolina AIDS Advisory Council. HIV/AIDS no longer posed such a threat to his friends: black heterosexuals and men who have sex with men (MSM) were more likely than white gays to acquire the virus in North Carolina; drug users and their sexual partners were at particular risk.[1] And the virus no longer spelled doom for those infected by it: within the previous year, protease inhibitors and Highly Active Anti-Retroviral Therapy (HAART) had cut AIDS mortality considerably. In December 1996, Jolly and his team released a report that prodded North Carolina to meet the chronic needs of people with AIDS.

By 1996, AIDS had dramatically transformed from the disease that first presented itself to Jolly and his colleagues over a decade earlier. The disease had become chronic and manageable, and activists, politicians, and health workers scrambled to find policies that would best control the epidemic. Finding "best policies," however, proved difficult, in part because various interest groups disagreed about what constituted "best" and in part because so many of the solutions still focused on individual behavior change. Since the AIDS epidemic flourished at the intersection of individual risk and sociostructural deficits, the individualist solutions did little to address the larger-scale structural issue that put groups of people at risk for HIV/AIDS. And since HIV/AIDS disproportionately affected African Americans, blacks in North Carolina continued to acquire HIV more frequently than the rest of the population, and their health fared worse once they got it. By the end of the 1990s, HIV/AIDS would become devastatingly endemic among African Americans in the state.

In 1996, the picture of AIDS in North Carolina was improved but still bleak. In December of that year, Jolly and his colleagues on the AIDS task force compiled an overview of the epidemic in the state. At that time, almost 10,000 North Carolinians were living with HIV. The mortality rate from AIDS was declining, which was excellent news, and the number of people diagnosed with HIV infection had also clearly fallen, although this last number was relative to the peak of new infections reported between 1992 and 1995 (part of this "spike" likely reflected new definitions, and better, more complete reporting of prevalent cases).[2] HIV infection remained a problem, however: the disease led causes of death for African American men aged fifteen to forty-four and was ranked as the second leading cause of death for African American females and of North Carolinians in general between those ages. More than 20 percent of new infections were coming from people aged twenty-five and younger. Ominously, in 1995, North Carolina had taken the lead among its neighboring states in the number of new and cumulative HIV infections.[3] HIV/AIDS continued to be a very real threat in North Carolina, exhibiting several worrying trends, and prevention remained essential to the fight.

AIDS therapy proved equally essential, of course, and in the 1990s patients and clinicians had a growing number of options from which to choose. At the same time, however, the growing burden of care associated with AIDS fell increasingly to states. This rendered people with AIDS vulnerable to whatever gaps, inefficiencies, and injustices existed in a state's health infrastructure. In North Carolina, state officials began buttressing the state's HIV care response in 1987. Legislators used federal funds to make AIDS drugs available to those lacking the means to pay for them on their own. In the first years of the program, legislators set eligibility criteria remarkably low, at only 85 percent of the federal poverty level (FPL).[4] Frequently, as Richard Rumley found in eastern North Carolina, this meant people with AIDS could qualify for Medicaid before they qualified for the state's drug assistance program, because the income eligibility levels for Medicaid were higher.[5] This was true even after the government made these drug assistance funds permanent through the Ryan White CARE Act's AIDS Drug Assistance Program (ADAP). By 1995, it had become clear that this eligibility level excluded a considerable number of the working poor and meant that people with AIDS and their families had to undergo profound economic devastation from the disease before they could qualify for medication assistance. So in 1995, legislators bumped eligibility up to 110 percent of the FPL, and two years later, they raised it again to 125 percent of the FPL.[6]

Though for many years the state had relied quite heavily on federal funds to address AIDS costs, in the early 1990s the growing epidemic forced lawmakers to add state money to the drug assistance program. Prior to 1993, North Carolina was one of only eleven states that did not spend any of its own dollars on AIDS care.[7] That year, legislators approved $200,000 to cover excess drug assistance costs, and they set aside an additional $500,000 for community-based AIDS organizations and AIDS foster care.[8] As AIDS cases climbed, drug resistance grew, and the antiviral repertoire expanded, North Carolina added to its "excess costs" budget: in 1995, the number jumped to $450,000 and in 1996 and 1997, the state earmarked $750,000.[9]

This influx of funds could barely keep up with existing needs, prompting David Jolly and the others on the AIDS Advisory Council to demand improvements in medical education, Medicaid funding mechanisms, and substance abuse prevention programs.[10] Moreover, with new drug regimens promising to transform HIV infection into a long-term chronic disease, the advisory council recommended that the state draft long-term strategies to address issues like drug addiction and catastrophic financial insurance.[11] Many North Carolina legislators were unprepared for or uninterested in such sweeping proposals, however.[12]

DESPITE THE SWEEPING NATURE of its recommendations, the advisory council as a whole remained optimistic about the future of the AIDS epidemic in North Carolina. This optimism stemmed largely from the impact that the newly released protease inhibitors and the therapies associated with them were having on HIV/AIDS mortality. Indeed, evidence that the new drug regimens were slashing HIV-related morbidity and mortality rates in the state was emerging even as the council wrote its report. By early 1997, HIV-related mortality in the state dropped by more than half. AIDS clinicians were cautiously optimistic. "Clearly, of the patients who come to our clinic, fewer are dying compared to last year," John Bartlett, director of Duke University Medical Center's infectious diseases clinic, told reporters in January 1997. "I think the potential is there to decrease [AIDS] as a leading cause of death."[13] "For the first time in a long time, many of us are feeling hopeful," concurred Evelyn Foust, director of AIDS prevention programs for the North Carolina Department of Health and Human Services (Foust had taken over for David Jolly in the AIDS control program).[14] Many were astounded at the impact of HAART. "It was like manna from heaven," Richard Rumley remembered. "Here we had people who were supposed to die, and we all thought they were supposed to die, but they were doing better and living. We were amazed."[15]

Patients experienced dramatic transformations. In January 1997, the

Blevins AIDS residence in Durham saw its first patient in eight years leave owing to improved health; and by May, Carrboro's AIDS residence had sent two patients home because of their recovered health.[16] One was former resident Terry Pierson. The thirty-four-year-old had moved into the house in 1996 expecting to die. His weight had dropped from 202 pounds to a skeletal 123, he had battled six different bouts of pneumonia in 1996 alone, and on two occasions he had been so weak that his doctors summoned his family because they doubted he would last the night. Then, in March 1997, Pierson's physicians put him on the HAART "cocktail," and the former carpenter responded immediately. In two months he had gained forty-five pounds and regained enough strength to move back in with his parents. "It's a different world," AIDS residence director Deb Young told reporters. "Right now, [Blevins House] sort of looks like a hotel; it used to look like a hospice."[17] "I was exhilarated," a Fayetteville man told reporters in 1997 after his "AIDS cocktail" generated similar results. "It was just the most wonderful feeling to know that I had been granted more time."[18]

HAART's success rate triggered speculation about an impending cure and stoked calls for earlier and more widespread testing. Several prominent media outlets began speculating whether HAART would transform the term "AIDS Crisis" into the term "AIDS Cure," while *Time* magazine christened David Ho, a leading HAART researcher and proponent, its "Man of the Year" for 1996.[19] Ho, who acknowledged that the drugs might not work for everyone, suggested at the 1996 International AIDS Conference in Vancouver, Canada, that therapies like HAART could theoretically eradicate HIV from the body.[20] Since HIV started working in the body right away, Ho maintained, clinicians should "hit HIV, early and hard," with HAART to keep HIV at almost unidentifiable levels.[21] By implication, of course, this meant that the United States needed to beef up its early testing efforts to identify newly infected people and immediately start them on a HAART regime; not only would this prevent HIV from ravaging their bodies, but it would keep viral counts so low that infected individuals would be much less likely to transmit the virus to others. HAART held huge promise both as a treatment and as preventive therapy.

While the funding influx improved access to AIDS therapies, it also pressured communities to coordinate their AIDS services so citizens could take advantage of these resources. In cities lacking lead agencies to coordinate such services, like Fayetteville, in Cumberland County, or Durham, in Durham County, people with HIV were left to navigate a patchwork of public and private service agencies on their own.[22] Neither city had the simple mechanisms to help residents obtain support to stay healthy and prevent further transmission. According to Fayetteville AIDS educator Ashley Rozier, the most help the majority of people with AIDS received in the mid-1990s was "a few minutes of counseling[,] and [then they were] sent on their way."[23] Billie Basket, a Cumberland County social worker who counseled people with HIV, concurred: "Basically, I have to tell these people that 'you've got the virus but until you get really, really sick there's not going to be anybody to help you.'" Observers in Durham County voiced similar complaints.[24]

Several factors conspired against service coordination. Cumberland County received a limited amount of federal and state AIDS funding, for example, but it then had to share that money with seven other counties. AIDS care and prevention needs easily outstripped the funds available. Organizational problems compounded the bureaucratic challenges. In 1994, for example, police arrested three of the local consortium staff for embezzling thousands of federal program dollars.[25] The consortium also lacked internal cohesion, as member-groups viewed each other competitively rather than collaboratively, and organizational differences split the group along racial and political lines.[26] These bureaucratic and organizational constraints hampered Fayetteville's ability to combat the epidemic's spread effectively or to provide a continuity of care for those living with HIV.

In rural communities, where services proved even scarcer, these coordination challenges only amplified the access issues faced by people with AIDS. Not many communities had physicians like Richard Rumley, who would use geographic information systems software to locate social services for patients. Many rural regions also lacked tertiary medical care facilities or HIV/AIDS clinics. By 1995, for example, only four of the ten counties in the Cape Fear region had designated AIDS clinics, despite the fact that HIV had spread to each of the counties (and many of the clinics that were available were open for only a half day each week).[27] The following year, North Carolina health officials acknowledged the growing needs in rural communities and established nine new HIV testing centers in nonmetropolitan areas. They believed these clinics would improve HIV surveillance and reduce the number of "functionally infectious" individuals in rural communities.[28] They also hoped the clinics could serve as hubs to improve rural residents' access to HIV care.[29] Reality proved more complicated, as Rumley well knew, because many residents of rural communities lacked health insurance, reliable transportation, and continuity in their health care. On top of this, the annual price tag for antiviral therapies, which frequently topped at $10,000 to $15,000, was well beyond the financial means of many rural people.[30] Often up to 30 percent of those with HIV in rural communities were uninsured and ineligible for Medicaid.[31] For many with HIV in rural communities, the increase in the number of HIV testing facilities did little to address the most glaring needs for managing their disease.

Under different circumstances, AIDS activists might have loudly confronted these gaps in care, but by the mid-1990s, middle-class white gays had largely achieved and were satisfied with the infrastructual supports they had sought from the system.[32] The normalization of AIDS meant that most AIDS care, control, and prevention took place within the mainstream health care infrastructure. Gay men and their allies in the AIDS advocacy community were largely responsible for bringing this about, but many of them were less attuned to the structural issues related to larger health disparities and the social determinants of health. And in the later 1990s, many of the communities being newly affected by HIV lacked a strong gay and lesbian community that would make AIDS a policy priority in those communities.[33] The demographic groups now being most affected by HIV/AIDS — injection drug users, those in their sexual networks, and minority MSM — lacked the comparable social capital or material resources to advocate on their own behalf.

Indeed, for many first-generation AIDS activists, the fight shifted in the 1990s to maintaining existing AIDS services and safeguarding existing AIDS policies. The effort that perhaps best symbolized this shift in priorities was the extended court battle that AIDS activists waged in the state to retain anonymous testing. As mentioned in previous chapters, North Carolina's Health Department decided to end anonymous testing in the state in 1990.[34] The phase-out began officially in July 1991, but ACT UP's legal team was able to block the new policy four months later.[35] The courts ruled that the phase-out plan had been "arbitrary and capricious," and when the state refused to reevaluate its policy, the court issued a permanent injunction against the policy in June 1993.[36]

These victories proved temporary, however. By 1993, the tide had clearly turned against anonymous testing: twenty-four states had already ended the practice, and the Centers for Disease Prevention and Control (CDC) recommended the others follow suit.[37] Moreover, data drawn from the period during which North Carolina had stopped anonymous testing in eighty-seven counties indicated that testing rates and HIV cases had remained stable and four times as many cases had been identified through contact tracing.[38] State health officials used this data to once again stop statewide anonymous testing in the summer of 1994, but ACT UP drew on some conflicting statistics to again secure a court injunction against the policy change.[39] The following year, the North Carolina Health Commission again outlawed anonymous testing, but ACT UP was able to launch an appeals process that prevented implementation of the regulations until the courts settled the matter.[40] Finally, in 1997, the courts ruled against ACT UP's complaint and removed all obstacles to the policy.[41] After a seven-year battle, North Carolina officially ended anonymous HIV testing in the state.

The changing nature of AIDS activism was mirrored in the 1990s with shifts in the constitution of AIDS Service Organizations. Whereas many AIDS organizations had been founded with an overtly gay identity, the mainstreaming of AIDS had diluted those commitments and the priorities that went with them. The Metrolina AIDS Project (MAP), for example, underwent internal battles over its identity that diluted some of the group's most pronounced gay characteristics (like staff and board makeup, program offerings, and care and prevention materials) and transformed it into a more traditional service provider. The issue came down to demographics: as the population affected by HIV changed, the organization eventually followed. "MAP looks nothing like what it did in 1984," David Jolly recalled. "Les Kooyman gets a lot of the credit. He took on his predominately gay white board and staff and said, 'Look, the epidemic is changing and we need to change. Look who our clients are. We need to be hiring African American people to work with our increasing African American client base.'"[42] MAP was able to transition from a support group for gay people with AIDS into a comprehensive AIDS Service Organization. Other groups, like the AIDS Services Agency of Wake County, likewise transitioned from being run largely by white gay men to being more aligned with the demographics of North Carolina's epidemic.[43]

Other groups were unable to make this transition, however. Durham's Lesbian and Gay Health Project (LGHP), for example, determined to preserve its homosexual identity. Relatively stable leadership allowed the group to survive and thrive in the lean economic times of the early 1990s, but in 1994 the limited funding and internal dissension left the group leaderless and adrift.[44] Consequently, the group collapsed. In 1994, the project had to cut back its support services due to funding constraints; and in June 1995, it lost its prevention grants and had to lay off its outreach workers.[45]

The demise of LGHP proved particularly troubling because it was allegedly the key AIDS Service Organization for the local Ryan White consortium. Between May and September of 1995, consortium staff repeatedly implored the LGHP to reinstate the services it had previously reined in. "The Consortium [has] shielded the Health Project from having to make big decisions about HIV service provision by supplying the illusion that service was being delivered," Piedmont Consortium director Susan Sachs wrote in May of that year.[46] "[There is a] dire need for coordinated, comprehensive HIV services in Durham," Sachs wrote again that September. "Literally hundreds of HIV+ Durham County residents with needs have to run the gamut in search of services and often, they are unable to get their needs met."[47] Ultimately, the LGHP proved unable to provide the services the Piedmont Consortium deemed essential, and the consortium itself began trying to meet the needs of people with AIDS in Durham County.[48] The LGHP, by now providing only a fraction of Durham's HIV services, was completely bypassed in the effort.[49] Although the group did hire a new director in the summer of 1995, the LGHP's financial and organizational situation proved too dysfunctional to repair and the director resigned less than three months later.[50] The group hobbled on for a few more months, but ultimately the effort proved unsustainable, and the group closed its doors. The entity that had shaped AIDS policy and pioneered AIDS service delivery in the state for over a decade had proved unable to weather the changing environment of AIDS funding and services, to adjust to the shifting demographics of the disease, or to establish local and regional funding streams that would have ensured the group's survival. By 1996, when David Jolly and the North Carolina AIDS Advisory Council drew up their list of active AIDS organizations in the state, the LGHP ceased to exist.[51]

AT THE SAME TIME these shifts in the focus of AIDS activists and the makeup of AIDS Service Organization occurred, sociopolitical conservatives were obtaining increasing control of many HIV/AIDS-related policies. AIDS activists and health officials had often battled the influence of sociopolitical conservatives both within and outside the administration during Republican governor Jim Martin's tenure (1985–93).[52] This fight only seemed to increase in 1994, after cultural conservatives gained control of the state legislature. Upon election, conservatives in the Republican Party began targeting things like abstinence education, passing the "Abstinence Until Marriage" bill in the summer of 1995.[53] The law required local school boards to institute an "abstinence until marriage" program by the 1996–97 school year. Responses to the law varied by county, in part because the legislation included a loophole that permitted school districts to sidestep more restrictive curriculum if they could gain parental support. So, in more conservative strongholds like Franklin County, in order to comply with the law, the school board hired a parent to tear three chapters out of the middle school health textbook. In more moderate Guilford County, the school board was able to obtain parental approval for a cautious but comprehensive sex education curriculum. And in Chapel Hill, a bastion of liberalism in the state, teachers openly taught middle school students about condom use and the ways that bleach killed HIV in contaminated needles.[54] Nonetheless, conservatives had been able to adjust the baseline sex education curriculum to the right, indicating yet another way that AIDS leadership and activism in the state was shifting away from its original sociopolitical makeup.

One final transition worth noting is that, by the mid-1990s, a growing number of African American groups took up the issue of HIV/AIDS. State efforts to reach African Americans had yielded few results. Several faith-based AIDS initiatives had sprung up in black communities to fill the gaps left by the state. As Janet Wise, assistant chief of the North Carolina Health Department's HIV/STD Control Section, put it in 1996, "I'm as black as your black shoes, but it won't do me any good to say that. I'm with the State. That's the system. It has to come from the ministers."[55] In 1995, 2,000 congregants participated in the annual "AIDS Sunday" outreach program in black churches. That same year, efforts by the American Red Cross to reach black pastors bore fruit when twenty-six Charlotte-area black churches launched new AIDS ministries.[56] In 1996, the CDC helped bring to North Carolina the "Black Church Week of Prayer for the Healing of AIDS," an initiative started in Harlem, New York, in 1989, to "mobilize the African-American religious community to address HIV/AIDS appropriately and effectively."[57] Black leaders and federal health officials had deemed the week of prayer so effective that the CDC worked in cooperation with state health departments to launch seven similar programs across the country; in 1996, Raleigh-Durham became one of those sites.[58] The program quickly spread to Gaston, Cumberland, and Mecklenburg counties.[59] Part of the program's attractiveness was that it sprang from the African American community itself and tackled AIDS in an appropriate cultural context. The program allowed churches to intervene on HIV/AIDS without their having to settle disagreements over the moral status of drug use, extramarital sex, and homosexuality.[60]

AIDS programs also sprang up in organizations outside black churches. By the mid-1990s, black Masons chapters, sickle cell organizations, black fraternities and sororities, and regional barbershop associations all began developing AIDS education programs. In Catawba County, a group of concerned black men launched a male-driven AIDS education program called Brothers United For Change.[61] Organizations like the African American Community

Endowment Fund, the Alpha Kappa Alpha Sorority, and the Sickle Cell Disease Association of the Piedmont all sponsored AIDS awareness programs in rural communities.[62] AIDS had finally gained a measure of traction and attention within North Carolina's African American community.

Still, the magnitude of the epidemic easily surpassed these mobilization efforts. By the mid-1990s, North Carolina had more new and cumulative HIV infections than Virginia, Tennessee, and South Carolina, and it rivaled only Virginia for total number of people with HIV/AIDS.[63] Meanwhile, rural counties continued to bear unprecedented burdens related to HIV, reporting some of the highest per capita HIV/AIDS rates in the state.[64] The ineffectiveness of prevention efforts in minority communities became acute at this time, as surveillance statistics indicated that African Americans constituted 77 percent of North Carolina's new HIV cases.[65] Moreover, when considered in relation to the proportion of the state population, African Americans in North Carolina were affected by HIV at rates higher than those in neighboring states.[66]

NOT ONLY DID African Americans lag behind other groups in the scope and effectiveness of prevention efforts, but as successful antiviral therapies became available, they found themselves trailing other groups in experiencing the benefits of those therapies in their communities. For example, when HAART became available in 1996, individuals without health insurance—a disproportionate number of whom were African Americans—had much more difficulty accessing these drugs.[67] Coverage gaps were most pronounced for those living with HIV in rural areas.[68] In North Carolina's Cape Fear region, for example, AIDS workers estimated that 90 percent of their clients were poor and that 95 percent lacked insurance.[69] The uninsured frequently postponed care until later in their disease progression, which increased their chances of passing the virus on and decreased their own survival rate.[70]

Even African Americans with insurance found it harder to access HAART when it first became available.[71] Many physicians who treated minorities lacked experience with HIV, so their patients were less likely to receive standard-of-care antiviral treatment or comorbidity prophylaxis. They were also more likely to undergo hospitalization and experienced worse survival outcomes than patients with experienced providers.[72] Even physicians experienced with HIV struggled with compliance concerns related to injection drug users, who were disproportionately minorities.[73] As mentioned above, the scarcity of AIDS-related medical services in rural counties compounded these access issues, even after the 1996 clinic upgrade.[74] It was not until 2000 that physicians in North Carolina were able to reduce substantially these therapeutic disparities.[75]

HAART compliance also influenced HIV outcomes among minorities. Transportation problems hampered many people from receiving consistent HIV care. In 1998, 30 percent of urban case managers and 58 percent of rural case managers considered transportation a "major problem" in treatment nonpersistence.[76] Transportation could be costly and cumbersome for any-one, and those in rural communities also had to travel large distances just to receive comprehensive and confidential AIDS care.[77]

Stigma also played a role. AIDS had elicited fear and discrimination from the epidemic's outset. Many, particularly those from small towns, kept their HIV status secret to avoid "discrimination, ridicule and embarrassment."[78] The most extreme example is Raleigh, a black gay man living in Guilford County, North Carolina, who so feared disclosure of his HIV status that he would travel several hours across the North Carolina mountains to visit Abraham Verghese's AIDS clinic in Johnston City, Tennessee.[79] Lori, a black woman interviewed by researcher Kate Whetten-Goldstein, felt so ostra-cized by her community because of her HIV status that she secluded herself. "I want[ed] to sit on the porch [but] I couldn't," she said, "'cause the people would come by and say, 'she got AIDS,' and even after I had [my son] and I started walking and getting out, it was like that. So I'm more of a person that stays secluded in. You don't see me out anymore, I don't party no more. I used to drink, get high. I don't do nothing no more, I just — it's like I'm secluding myself."[80] Lisa, another North Carolinian interviewed by Whetten-Goldstein, was warned by her infected boyfriend not to reveal her HIV status to her mother. "Don't you [tell your mother], don't you tell nobody!" he said. "She'll hate you for the rest of your life!"[81] Gina, who was also interviewed by Whetten-Goldstein, stopped seeing one of her care providers because he suggested that she lose weight (to improve her overall health). She was afraid weight loss would reveal her HIV status to her friends. "I got this theory if you lose all that weight, then everybody is gonna know you are sick because they are going to say, 'Ooh, you done lost all that weight; you must be sick with the AIDS virus.'"[82] Although stigma did not prevent these people from care, it did make them — and countless others like them — less likely to adhere to their treatment recommendations. People with HIV/AIDS in North Carolina, especially in rural settings, frequently would skip doses when they were in public to avoid disclosing their HIV status.[83] Case managers in North Carolina reported that HIV-related stigma reduced adherence among patients in both urban (35 percent) and rural (92 percent) settings.[84]

Perceived side effects from the AIDS drugs also encouraged treatment non-compliance. Joni, a black woman in Whetten-Goldstein's study, said that HIV medications discolored and coarsened her skin and left her lethargic and in unbearable pain. "Sometimes I just lay in there like my bones aching," she told Whetten-Goldstein's team. "[My] skin is changing. I got this constant cough. . . . I always got a sinus infection. It is affecting my vision. Seems like my ears hurt. My whole body hurts. I just don't feel well ever, and I told you I stopped taking the pills, right. The pills don't make me feel no better."[85] Worried that others would notice what she believed to be side effects of drug therapy and discover her HIV status, Joni stopped taking her medication. Likewise Barb, the woman from Charlotte discussed in chapter 5, frequently failed to take her medications because of side effects she ascribed to the drugs. "AZT slows me down," Barb told a reporter. "When I don't take it, I can clean this house. It causes me bad headaches and side effects I can't handle, mood changes I can't handle. I get angry with my children."[86] Barb's and Joni's reasons for discontinuing their drug treatment proved all too common among people with HIV.

Other factors, including discontinuous care, inadequate housing, untreated substance abuse, and lack (or unawareness) of support services, led to treatment noncompliance. Indeed, the experience of HIV often seemed like just one additional problem in a lifetime of tragic struggle; noncompliance often indicated that people with HIV/AIDS felt much more pressing concerns than the management of a long-term chronic infection.[87]

THE CHALLENGES AIDS POSED to North Carolina had been playing out in similar ways in other southeastern states since the beginning of the epidemic. In the early part of the twenty-first century, southern states accounted for seven of the ten states with the highest AIDS case rates in the country.[88] HIV among young adults was disproportionately concentrated in the South. AIDS incidence (the number of newly diagnosed cases) continued rising in the American southeast between 1996 and 2001, even as it declined or remained constant in other parts of the country.[89] By 2002, the South had caught up to the rest of the country in terms of percentage of people living with HIV/AIDS (40 percent of HIV cases versus 38 percent of the U.S. population), but it accounted for 46 percent of new cases, suggesting that the epidemic had shifted toward the South.[90] Eighteen of the twenty-five metropolitan areas with an above average number of AIDS cases were located in the South, as were "6 of the metropolitan areas with the 10 highest AIDS case rates."[91] As in North Carolina, cases across the South disproportionately affected African Americans.

In light of these trends, in 2001, AIDS directors from southern states formed a work group as part of the National Alliance of State and Territorial AIDS Directors. Evelyn Foust, head of North Carolina's HIV/STD Prevention and Care Branch, served as a co-chair of the work group, and three other staffers served the unit as well.[92] The group met in Nashville in early 2002 to begin work on a "Call to Action" addressing the problem of AIDS in the American South. In November of that year, in collaboration with interested researchers, foundations, community activists, and other government entities, the group presented a draft manifesto to the Southern States Summit on HIV/AIDS and STDs, which met in Charlotte. "North Carolina is here today," explained Steven Cline, the head of North Carolina's division of epidemiology, "because . . . our HIV/AIDS and STD rates continue to increase . . . [and] they are disproportionately affecting a number of our citizens."[93] "The HIV/AIDS epidemic . . . is especially troubling for the southern region," noted Drew Altman, president and CEO of the Kaiser Family Foundation, a key sponsor of the summit. "By bringing these key groups together to strategize on combating HIV/AIDS and STDs in the southern United States, we hope to be able to make great strides towards reducing the disproportionate effects of these epidemics on minority Americans."[94] "This summit . . . is not just another meeting," Foust explained. "We're here to talk about what we will do. . . . This summit is a call for action. It's a call to synthesize our determination, our expertise so that the Southern people that we represent and the Southern people that we serve can live healthier lives."[95]

Formally released in March 2003, the "Southern States Manifesto" drew attention to the disproportionate number of newly diagnosed HIV infections in the South, the impact of AIDS on minority communities, and the inequitable regional distribution of federal funds (through the Ryan White CARE Act) in light of the burden of AIDS in the South.[96] The document laid out the various barriers to HIV/AIDS funding, leadership, partnerships, health equity, infrastructure, and state involvement, and provided specific action points to remove them.[97] The AIDS directors highlighted the problems of poverty, disparity in health care access, and poor health care infrastructure in the South that exacerbated the epidemic, and expressed considerable frustration at the Ryan White CARE Act's underfunding, particularly in the money it devoted to prevention and the methods by which it disbursed funds regionally. Motivated by the issues raised at these various conferences, a group of stakeholders formally launched the Southern AIDS Coalition (SAC), a membership organization of concerned parties willing to draw attention to and advocate on behalf of "the needs presented by the epidemics of HIV/AIDS and STDs in the southern United States."[98]

Admittedly, SAC members were playing catch-up. The epidemic continued to take its toll in the South in the ensuing years. Between 2001 and 2005, for example, the number of deaths attributable to AIDS dropped in the rest of the country but continued to rise in the South.[99] In 2005, half of all U.S. deaths from AIDS occurred in the South.[100] The South now boasted the highest number of adults and adolescents living and dying with the disease. State health care systems became increasingly overwhelmed by the growing caseload, and the number of those affected easily outstripped the resources available.[101] In large measure, the structural challenges that enabled HIV/AIDS to flourish in southern minority communities—high levels of STIs, lower levels of overall health, and elevated levels of socioeconomic vulnerability—continued unabated.[102] And the epidemic in the South continued to affect a more diverse, less urbanized, population than in other parts of the country.[103] Equally important was the rise of HIV/AIDS among Latinos: by 2006, HIV/AIDS was disproportionately affecting Latinos in the United States, as it was in the South.[104]

In light of these trends, SAC members criticized federal AIDS funding priorities.[105] In 2005, total CDC and Ryan White funding failed to reflect the disproportionate impact AIDS was having on the South. Despite bearing the greatest burden of active disease and new infections of any region in the country, and although trailing only the Northeast in number of AIDS cases per 100,000 people, the South received the smallest share of total federal and CDC HIV/AIDS funds than any region in the country. Only Ryan White funds—which ranked second in funding amounts by region per person living with AIDS—were commensurate with the number of cases in the South.[106] One of SAC's major efforts in the years after its launch was "to advocate for increased federal funding for prevention, treatment, care, and housing to rectify the historical inequities embedded in the federal HIV and STD funding portfolios."[107] SAC members were actively involved in the federal "discussions and negotiations that resulted in the passage of" the Ryan White HIV/AIDS Treatment Modernization Act (RWHATMA) of 2006.

As mentioned in chapter 5, the original Ryan White legislation addressed resource deficiencies in communities most impacted by HIV/AIDS. Throughout the 1990s and early 2000s, as the epidemic moved beyond its initial epicenters, health officials in increasingly affected regions began raising objections to constraints inherent in the legislation. SAC members in particular had several complaints about the program. First, they believed the CARE Act was "significantly underfunded," given that it reached twice as many people as Medicaid but received only a quarter of the funds.[108] Second, since patients diagnosed in urban centers frequently returned for care to their rural hometowns, SAC advocates felt CARE's funding structure overemphasized the place of diagnosis (often coastal/northern cities) and neglected locations of care (often southern/rural communities), to the detriment of the latter.[109] Third, they felt the program funds available to hard-hit cities (known as Title I) privileged northern and coastal regions with large cities and high numbers of AIDS cases. Title I had originally directed funds to Eligible Metropolitan Areas (EMA), which the CARE Act designated as cities with populations over 500,000. The South had fewer cities with populations greater than 500,000, but eventually it had higher numbers of people living with AIDS than other parts of the country with big cities. (In 2005, for example, the South reported 169,972 cases, versus 126,867 in the Northeast, 83,405 in the West, and 45,666 in the Midwest.)[110] SAC members advocated changes in the Ryan White CARE Act "so that funding follows the epidemic."[111]

The RWHATMA addressed many of these concerns by making the law more flexible to the changing epidemic. A revised distribution methodology made Part A/Title I funds more accessible to southern communities by reducing EMA size requirements down to 50,000. Eligibility and funding mechanisms were redesigned to include HIV cases and living AIDS cases, making the legislation more responsive to the shape of the epidemic in the South. The legislation also made more money and resources available to affected communities and established baseline drug and core services guidelines. Though SAC members appreciated many of these improvements, they felt the changes remained inadequate to meet the larger needs generated by the epidemic, especially since federal funding "failed to provide increases in prevention, care, treatment, and housing."[112]

At the same time that the government was revising the Ryan White legislation, the CDC released its "Revised Recommendations for HIV Testing of Adults, Adolescents, and Pregnant Women in Health-Care Settings."[113] The CDC's recommendations on HIV counseling and testing had evolved over the years in response to the changing epidemic and to political pressures and professional opinion. Initially, the CDC had stressed anonymous counseling and testing owing to professional divisions over what a positive antibody test meant, how cost effective it was versus other strategies, and how useful it was for patients in the absence of effective treatment. As the meaning of test results became clearer over the next years, the CDC expanded its recommendations for targeted HIV testing.[114] In 1987, it recommended "routine" voluntary testing for high-risk individuals, in 1993 it called for voluntary counseling and testing in hospitals and outpatient settings, and in 1995 it called for the testing of pregnant women. Beginning in 2001, the CDC unfolded a series of guidelines that made HIV testing easier and more routine in most health care settings. These culminated in the 2006 guidelines, which called for "routine HIV screening of adults, adolescents, and pregnant women in health care settings" in order to "reduc[e] barriers to HIV testing."[115] SAC members welcomed these revised recommendations, considering them "essential in the South." Since the South was "the fastest growing region [in the country] for new HIV infections," SAC participants felt that "the implementation of these guidelines would result in a reduction of new infections, . . . protect unborn infants of HIV-positive mothers . . . [and] greatly increase the opportunity for persons to learn of their status."[116]

While SAC members considered these policy changes and recommendations important in the fight against AIDS in the South, they also recognized that without leadership and political will, the South would not get the full benefit from them. Consequently, in SAC's *Southern States Manifesto: Update 2008*, they called on policymakers and state health officials to work together to reduce late-term AIDS diagnoses; increase HIV, STD, or hepatitis status awareness; increase "age-appropriate, science-driven education"; improve health outcomes for people with HIV/AIDS; implement the CDC opt-out testing recommendations; increase outreach and access to HIV counseling, testing, and screening; and increase state and federal funding "for prevention, treatment, care, housing, and services for people living with or at risk of HIV/AIDS, STDs, and hepatitis."[117] As the U.S. presidential election season geared up, they turned their attention to the growing push for health care reform that was coming from the candidates in 2008.[118]

The policy changes also had an important impact on the management of HIV in North Carolina. In October 2006, through the activism of Evelyn Foust and other AIDS allies in the state, North Carolina launched an "aggressive statewide HIV screening initiative" called "Get Real. Get Tested."[119] The initiative combined high-visibility radio, television, and print media ads with door-to-door community campaigns and community-based mobile testing efforts.[120] "Get Real. Get Tested" increased HIV testing by over 18 percent in one year through its combination of broad messaging and nontraditional targeted testing.[121]

Foust and her allies were also able to convince lawmakers to increase ADAP financial eligibility from 125 to 250 percent of the federal poverty level. Eventually, state lawmakers pushed that number to 300 percent of FPL. "That [was] huge," Foust told reporters in December 2009. "That was our hard fought battle to [get] North Carolina to the national average. . . . We, in the past, had waiting lists, today we are open, we are serving people that could not otherwise access these medications. So it's been a huge success."[122] Unfortunately, the recession of 2009 hit state finances hard, and, in the summer of 2009, the General Assembly approved a bill that cut more than $3 million from the state's ADAP program. Beginning in January of 2010, the state began putting new applicants on a waiting list. The budget proposed later that spring offered to reinstate the program, but it reduced eligibility back down to its pre-2006 level of 125 percent of FPL.[123] Despite the setbacks on drug access predicted for 2010, the availability of HAART for people with HIV was having an important impact on life with the disease. Like many other states, North Carolina saw extraordinary reductions in HIV-associated morbidity and mortality after the introduction of protease inhibitor–based HAART. In 1993, the average time between diagnosis of HIV and the diagnosis of AIDS was 2.8 years; in 2008 the average had climbed to 7.2 years.[124] More people were living with, rather than dying from, HIV/AIDS in the state. HIV had truly become a chronic, manageable disease in North Carolina.[125]

While HIV infection had become a manageable disease, it nonetheless continued spreading throughout the state. Indeed, beginning in 2001, the number of reported HIV cases again began creeping upward: annual reported cases topped 1,600 in 2002 and surpassed 2,000 by 2006; only the four years immediately preceding the use of protease inhibitors had seen higher annual caseloads.[126] While some of the increases likely stemmed from "newly implemented surveillance activities that added some older prevalent cases to the system," the increase (or absence of a decline) nevertheless remained disheartening.[127]

The demographics of these new cases were changing, too. MSM remained the principal mode of infection transmission (51 percent of cases reported), with heterosexual transmission following close behind (40 percent of cases reported). The balance seemed to be shifting within these categories, however, for whereas in 2002, MSM constituted 59 percent of new infections, by 2006 they made up 71 percent of new cases. By 2006, injection drug users constituted only 6 percent of cases reported.[128] Within these categories there was considerable variability, however. Among white males, MSM accounted for 86 percent of reported cases, heterosexuals about 8 percent, and intravenous drug users about 3 percent. Among black males, MSM made up 63 percent of reported cases, heterosexuals, about 30 percent, and intravenous drug users, about 5 percent. Among other minority groups (Hispanics, American Indians, and Asian/Pacific Islanders), who constituted a smaller number of cases, 61 percent of reported cases among men were MSM, 29 percent were heterosexual, and 7 percent were intravenous drug users.[129] North Carolina's epidemic was also becoming an increasingly rural phenomenon. In 2003, more than 25 percent of AIDS reports in North Carolina came from nonmetropolitan areas. Only one other state in the nation reported higher nonmetropolitan numbers at that time, and only four other states reported as many nonmetropolitan HIV cases (that is, non-AIDS).[130]

Problematically, many of these newly infected individuals were discovering their infection late in the progression of their illness. Even after the various outreach efforts had been implemented, anywhere from 30 to 50 percent of new HIV cases reported each year were also recorded as new AIDS cases.[131] Between 2004 and 2008, more than half the AIDS diagnoses in the state came from people at late stages of HIV infection (AIDS was the initial diagnosis or it was "diagnosed within 6 months of the initial HIV diagnosis").[132] Since early diagnosis prevented new HIV infections ("knowledge of positive HIV status promotes adoption of safer sex practices") and those testing late were more likely to develop AIDS (they only partially benefited from antiretroviral therapy and comorbidity prophylaxis), the large number of late diagnoses served only to further the virus's spread while imposing greater socioeconomic burdens on individuals, their families, and the state.[133]

Finally, the racial disparities in HIV transmission rates remained. The rate of infection for non-Hispanic blacks was eight times higher than for non-Hispanic whites; black men had rates seven times higher than white men, and black women had rates seventeen times higher than non-Hispanic white women.[134] The disparity in AIDS rates was even higher: blacks had ten times the rate for whites and over twice the rate for Hispanics.[135] Moreover, this rate was increasing. Between 2004 and 2008, the AIDS case rate climbed 19 percent among black women and 8 percent among black men. In 2007, HIV disease was the third leading cause of death for women aged twenty-five to forty-four and the fourth leading cause of death for black men in the same age category.[136] In 2008, minorities accounted for 78 percent of new AIDS cases diagnosed in the state (blacks, 69 percent; Hispanics, 8 percent; Caucasians, 22 percent).[137] Hispanics, too, were seeing dramatic increases. Between 2004 and 2008, the rate of AIDS diagnosis had increased 115 percent. AIDS cases had jumped 139 percent among Hispanic males (from 10.5

to 25.1 per 100,000) and 43 percent among Hispanic females (from 4.2 to 6.0 per 100,000). Given the migratory nature of some Hispanic communities, these figures are estimates, but they still outstripped the estimated population growth of Hispanic communities in North Carolina, which increased an estimated 34 percent between 2004 and 2008.[138] Consequently, Hispanics had an AIDS case rate four times higher than Caucasians in North Carolina, and among adults aged twenty-five to forty-four, HIV disease stood as the fourth leading cause of death for Hispanic females and the tenth leading cause of death for Hispanic males in 2007.[139]

People involved in AIDS prevention and treatment, like Evelyn Foust in the Department of Health's Communicable Disease Branch, were therefore under no illusions about the severity of the situation as North Carolina approached the end of the third decade of the AIDS epidemic. They continued "actively pursuing new policies and guidelines" to include HIV testing in "routine medical care settings." They also continued pushing to expand rapid HIV testing in "nontraditional and high prevalence settings." And they stressed programs like their "Get Real. Get Tested" campaign to prompt North Carolinians to get tested.[140] Still, with budget cuts looming in the wake of the recession of the late 2000s, they knew conditions could easily grow worse. Foust and her colleagues had made profound strides against HIV in North Carolina, but they still had miles to go.

WATSON AND THE SHARK

The Past and Future of AIDS in North Carolina
and the American South

At the end of a long hall in Washington D.C.'s National Gallery of Art hangs John Singleton Copley's *Watson and the Shark*. The eighteenth-century painting depicts a young sailor being attacked by a shark while his crewmates struggle mightily to beat back the shark and save him. Art historians tell us that the painting was inspired by a real event in Havana, Cuba, in 1749, when fourteen-year-old Brook Watson was attacked by a shark in the Havana harbor. An orphan serving as a crew member on a trading ship, Watson was swimming alone in the harbor when he was attacked, and his shipmates—men of various ethnic backgrounds and social stations— immediately launched a heroic effort to save him. Brook Watson survived the attack, and after having his leg amputated below the knee, went on to become, among other things, an English baron and the lord mayor of London. Watson himself commissioned the painting from his friend Copley.[1]

As Richard Rumley journeyed through counties of eastern North Carolina, pleading with various citizen groups not to ignore HIV/AIDS, he carried a copy of Copley's *Watson and the Shark*. "When [Copley] did it, it was to symbolize community spirit: government and citizens working together for a common cause," Rumley explained. "So I used that in my talks, and tried to help with that." Rumley would conclude his talk with Matthew 25:40 and an impassioned call to action. "I was trying to get them to realize that . . . the thing that tells people that they're all the same is the pain and suffering that they deal with and that they try to fix as a community. Like my Watson and the Shark picture . . . that's what brings people together. Yeah, it's a terrible disease and it does terrible things to people, but it brings people together. It should, anyway. And I think one day it will bring people together. But I think it's just a long time in the making."[2]

INDEED, NORTH CAROLINA'S HIV epidemic was a long time in the making, and, at the time of this writing, it continues. In the early years of the epidemic, when the state ranked twenty-third in the number of new AIDS cases diagnosed, few observers would have imagined that by 2007 North Carolina would climb into the top ten states in this regard.[3] Yet that has been the trajectory of the epidemic in North Carolina. The epidemic's course mirrors that in other states in many ways: the first cases appeared in the late 1970s and early 1980s, and it disproportionately affected white and black men who have sex with men (MSM) and black intravenous drug users. HIV among white MSM climbed rapidly in the 1980s, plateaued by the early 1990s, and declined thereafter to a stable baseline. HIV among black MSM, intravenous drug users, and their partners likewise rose rapidly in the 1980s, surpassing Caucasians by 1988, and continued climbing into the mid-1990s. While the number of new cases dropped in the second half of the 1990s, they began climbing again in the early 2000s, as HIV proliferated among black MSM and heterosexuals and in impoverished rural communities. As this study makes clear, North Carolina's HIV epidemic disproportionately affected African Americans from the very beginning, and those trends have only grown worse.

At various times throughout the epidemic, regional and national observers have discussed the "changing face of AIDS," that is, it initially predominantly affected white gay men but increasingly affected women and minorities. In the South, and in North Carolina in particular, however, HIV always disproportionately affected African Americans. In North Carolina and much of the South, activists and health workers were able to rein in the epidemic among white MSM, while the disease continued to flourish among black MSM and intravenous drug users and spread into other black sexual networks. For white gay males in North Carolina, advocates and health workers were largely able to identify the factors driving the epidemic and implement care and prevention strategies that brought the epidemic under some measure of control. African Americans, whether male or female, gay or straight, urban or rural, were not so fortunate.

The story of AIDS in white communities and the story of AIDS in African American communities are quite different, but they also intersect. On its own, the story of white gay men in the South is an important story to tell, of course, and historians need to do more work exploring the emergence of white AIDS organizations in the American South. The story of the Lesbian and Gay Health Project (LGHP) in Durham needs to be supplemented with the story of AIDS activists in Atlanta and Houston, if only to expand our understanding of AIDS activism beyond that gleaned from the traditional narrative of activists in New York, California, and Washington, D.C. Some of this work is just now being done. But the story of white AIDS organizations in the South is also important because white gay men there frequently became advocates for other marginalized groups who were vulnerable to HIV. As AIDS clinician Charles van der Horst noted in a 1998 interview, "The gay community in North Carolina has been unbelievable. . . . It would be like during World War II asking the Jews to say, 'Okay, I want you to be a self-help organization, but I want you to help the Gypsies too, and the gays that are being annihilated.' [Gays in North Carolina have been] willing to do that."[4] Gay men, lesbians, and their allies in southern AIDS organizations frequently became the main advocates speaking out for the individuals and families being decimated by HIV.

White gay organizations had a limited impact on the HIV epidemic, however, because the social worlds of white and black MSM rarely intersected, largely mirroring the functional segregation of the races in the state. Consequently, white gay groups like the LGHP had little contact with minority gays and even less influence over any protective behaviors they might adopt. Moreover, the outreach and prevention strategies championed by white AIDS organizations targeted middle-class white gays. They therefore had limited effect even among rural, blue-collar, and non-gay-identified white men, to say nothing of the poor, rural, and non-gay-identifying blacks. Targeting gay bars, for example, proved insufficient in places where few bars existed for black gays. Since white gay men strongly supported the voluntary ethic embodied in AIDS exceptionalism, their inability to reach black MSM cast doubts on the suitability of this approach as a long-term policy solution in North Carolina.

While white gays played an important role in the formulation and implementation of HIV policy in North Carolina, this should not be confused with culpability. The reality is that black MSM themselves were ineffective in encouraging and sustaining substantive behavior change. African American men are not strictly unusual in this respect: adopting and sustaining protective sexual behaviors has proved difficult for most people.[5] But several factors hindered these behaviors among black MSM in North Carolina. Perhaps most importantly, many black men did not consider themselves at risk for HIV infection. Many of Garry Lipscomb's contacts, for example, believed HIV to be a disease one acquired by having sex with white men, and none of them had sex with white men. Ignorance about their individual risk left many black men unprepared to deal with HIV. In addition, black MSM lacked an externally visible community in North Carolina, that is, many did not self-identify as gay or had yet to "come out" to the extent that many white gays had. Consequently, African Americans in North Carolina had neither the broadly based network of resources that enabled white gay communities to organize around AIDS nor the indigenous care and prevention structures that came with them. Thus, while it is likely that most black MSM supported the privacy considerations of AIDS exceptionalism, the community proved unable to generate a compensatory level of AIDS awareness necessary for it to succeed among black MSM. Moreover, other groups could not offset these gaps in indigenous AIDS organizing.

Indeed, black health organizations in general faced similar limitations reaching black MSM. The contested place of homosexuality in the African American community meant that many of these organizations had little contact with black MSM. Homonegativity in black communities—especially in black churches—served to buttress the larger cultural efforts by social conservatives to stigmatize homosexual behavior. Black MSM in North Carolina existed largely "underground." Moreover, with black men underrepresented in the health profession, black health organizations lacked the connections and credibility with black MSM necessary to reach them effectively. Frequently, groups like Howard Fitts's AIDS Clearinghouse concentrated on black drug users, hoping that white AIDS organizations would be better positioned to reach black MSM. Since AIDS exceptionalism kept HIV testing voluntary and nonroutine, an at-risk black MSM could pass through numerous points within North Carolina's health system over several years without ever receiving HIV education or undergoing HIV testing. Black MSM existed at those social interstices where homophobia had marginalized them, AIDS groups (black and white) could not effectively reach them, and AIDS exceptionalism made it very difficult for them to be "found."

Since Rebecca Meriwether and David Jolly relied so heavily on community-based AIDS organizations to implement AIDS care and prevention efforts in affected communities, it is not difficult to understand why state outreach efforts proved relatively ineffective in their endeavor to reach black MSM. Added to this was the fact that the public health community lacked, and still largely lacks, prevention models of proven effectiveness among black MSM.[6] Conflating behavioral risks (for example, anal receptive sex) with social identity ("gay," "straight," or "bisexual") obfuscated the heterogeneity of values, identities, and resources within those broad categories. This, in turn, had important implications for the effectiveness of outreach and intervention, not to mention research design.[7]

This problem clearly also has important implications for understanding the history of AIDS beyond North Carolina or the American South. On top of this, of course, the state's AIDS control program rarely had enough time, staff, or resources to explore risk behaviors effectively or design culturally tailored, evidence-based interventions to address them. Consequently, even if AIDS Service Organizations and county health departments had been sufficiently staffed and resourced, they would still have lacked prevention efforts with proven effectiveness for North Carolina's risk populations.

The struggles that North Carolina's AIDS prevention programs encountered had important implications for effective outreach to sexual minorities. As Ford et al. have noted, basing prevention strategies on rigid conceptualizations of sexual identity will overlook the fluid nature of sexuality in marginalized communities.[8] The success of outreach among white gay communities in North Carolina was based on their widespread involvement in the formulation and implementation of those strategies in their communities; the lack of similar participation among black MSM at almost every level in North Carolina can not be ignored when judging the ineffectiveness of those outreach efforts. In North Carolina's case, relying on "persons with less social distance from the target population" did not prove as effective as desired.[9] Prevention systems that lack redundancy, providing a monophonic rather than a polyphonic outreach strategy, will fail when applied to doubly marginalized groups.[10] In North Carolina's case, even when health professionals "triangulated" their prevention efforts (utilizing both black and gay groups to reach black MSM), their efforts met with failure. Health systems must include primary target populations in the research, planning, and implementation of outreach efforts and buttress those with multiple levels of redundant prevention systems to ensure those already "underground" or at greatest risk for "falling through the cracks" can, in fact, effectively be reached.[11]

Reaching sexual communities was only part of the problem. Prevention efforts among drug addicts, a majority of whom were minorities, proved equally difficult. Little self-organizing around harm reduction occurred in North Carolina. People like Harold Burton, the Durham man who, after his AIDS diagnosis, began warning his former needle-sharing partners about their risks for the disease, proved the exception rather than the rule. Moreover, the addiction rehabilitation community failed to understand the threat that HIV posed to its clientele for much of the 1980s. Some addiction programs, like Project Straighttalk in Durham, did create interventions for drug users (including bleach kits and needle exchange programs), but North Carolina provided insufficient funds for addiction-related health services, and efforts remained few and far between. Additionally, many of the prevention efforts concentrated on shared needles among injection drug users, while a substantial portion of the drug problem that fueled HIV transmission in North Carolina centered on cocaine and crack cocaine and the transactional sex related to them. North Carolina's meager commitment to mental health and addiction services left many people vulnerable to these risks.

Underestimating complex behavioral connections—like those between noninjection drug use and risky transactional sex—was not solely a problem of the substance abuse community. As Richard Rumley recognized in the early 1990s, HIV transmission depended on a host of sociostructural factors endemic to North Carolinian society. Migration patterns, economic conditions, and incarceration policies played an important role incentivizing concurrent sexual partnerships and risky sexual behaviors so that black women and rural minorities unwittingly became exposed to HIV. The majority of public health strategies against HIV in North Carolina located the cause of HIV in individuals and their risky lifestyle behaviors, a perspective that proved insufficient to address the larger sociocultural pathways that led to HIV acquisition and progression. Likewise, the personal privacy concerns of largely middle-class gay communities came to dominate AIDS strategies adopted by AIDS exceptionalists. People concerned that anything other than voluntary anonymous testing (that is, "opt-in," "opt-out," "routine," or "provider-initiated" testing schemas) might drive high-risk people "underground" failed to ensure that compensatory measures were put in place to reach those members of society who, owing to a host of sociostructural factors, already lacked access to the system or who were unaware of their own risk. Conversely, many social and political conservatives who demanded coercive public health measures failed to recognize that those measures alone had not curbed the epidemic in other states. Name-based testing, on its own, had not necessarily slowed the epidemic in southern states. A much broader-based investment in the social determinants of HIV was needed to control the epidemic. With AIDS then, as with many diseases, both sides of the social contract needed to be upheld for interventions to work. Individual responsibility to society and society's responsibility to at-risk individuals depended on each other.[12]

The history of HIV in North Carolina highlights both the strengths and weaknesses of the state's health system. The state's public and private hospitals began providing care for people with HIV very early in the epidemic. Indeed, UNC cared for its first AIDS patient the same month that the Centers for Disease Control and Prevention reported the first AIDS cases. By 1986, state health officials had set up HIV counseling and testing facilities in every county, had established a collaborative relationship with AIDS activists in gay communities, and had hired the state's most prominent AIDS organizer, David Jolly, to spearhead the state AIDS program. Each of these leadership decisions ensured that North Carolina was well-positioned to respond effectively, flexibly, and appropriately to the epidemic as health officials understood it. This was an important feat in a conservative state. State and local health workers also responded rapidly to the opportunities presented to them in the early 1990s with the advent of the Ryan White CARE Act and the success of Highly Active Antiretroviral Therapy (HAART).

On the other hand, AIDS care and prevention in North Carolina also suffered from several limitations. State investment in AIDS care proved mediocre, particularly when compared with that of nearby states. Poor or insufficient surveillance often prevented state and local health professionals from following the epidemic as it moved into new areas or populations. Rural communities suffered in this regard, and even patients in urban areas lacked sufficient continuity of care. For many observers, North Carolina's Medicaid eligibility requirements were tragically restrictive, forcing many to impoverish themselves just to qualify for help and leaving many others on waiting lists owing to financial constraints and restrictions. On top of this, federal formulations for funding distribution underestimated the nature and severity of the epidemic in the South and consequently underfunded, and continue to underfund, HIV care and prevention efforts in places like North Carolina. Finally, the constant political interplay with social conservatives kept state and local health workers from implementing effective, evidence-based HIV intervention programs for various target groups (that is, by risk category or age range).

Social conservatives and conservative social policy cannot be disregarded here, although both have served mostly as a backdrop in this study. Still, two aspects of their influence deserve attention. First, AIDS policy in North Carolina was forged in and responded to a socially conservative culture. As members of a sexual minority, gay men in North Carolina found their collective legitimacy and social acceptance under constant threat, and social conservatives represented the key embodiment of that threat. Gay men had endured years of overt and covert discrimination in North Carolina: anti-gay and AIDS-related discrimination rose during the 1980s and 1990s, and in the early 1990s, North Carolina actually led the country in the number of anti-gay hate crimes reported. Accordingly, gay men and their allies specifically framed their HIV care and prevention strategies with those real and perceived threats in mind. Perhaps the most obvious example of this, the struggle for anonymous testing and contact tracing, was forged in this context. Social conservatives therefore represented both real and symbolic antagonists, in response to which the AIDS exceptionalist alliance forged their AIDS policies.

While it is inappropriate to conflate all homonegative actions with social conservatives, some social conservatives truly did serve as opponents in the AIDS policy debate. State representative Coy Privette and his legislative allies, for example, sought to constrain the content and extent of publicly supported HIV education and outreach, particularly in the public school curriculum, and David Jolly met similar opposition within North Carolina's public health infrastructure. Even where social conservatives did recommend potentially effective public health interventions (name-based HIV testing and contact tracing, for example), their versions of those policies tended to be highly coercive and punitive, and they were often bundled with inappropriate and ineffective interventions (such as food service restrictions or mandatory premarital testing, for example). Moreover, social conservatives served as the main opposition to North Carolina's antidiscrimination laws. Research indicates that both enacted stigma (active discrimination based on moral, social, racial, or physical "taint") and felt stigma (the fear or experience of enacted stigma) serve as barriers to surveillance of and treatment for a host of diseases, including HIV.[13] Thus, even when social conservatives proposed policies that might have improved North Carolina's HIV surveillance, prevention, and control, their resistance to the active protection of citizens from discrimination or to insurance safeguards eroded the very trust and cooperation on which those policies depended. Moreover, their role in cultivating enacted or felt AIDS-related stigma makes them culpable for (at least) that component of the epidemic. As Ronald Bayer has argued, preventing the spread of HIV depended on a reciprocal relationship between health officials and those at risk of infection and transmission; both needed to participate in a "culture of responsibility" if such efforts were to be effective.[14] In North Carolina, social conservatives demanded that those at risk for HIV adopt a culture of responsibility, but, when it came to policy, they failed to provide the reciprocal commitments and protections.

WHAT LARGER RELEVANCE does the history of the AIDS epidemic in North Carolina have? Clearly, each state has its own story, but that does not make each story equally valuable to understanding the larger history of HIV in the United States. Any historian would argue that every story is worth telling on its own merits, but beyond that, the story of AIDS in North Carolina touches on several important themes that help fill out the larger history of HIV in America.

The most obvious purpose this study serves is to draw attention to the true shape of the AIDS epidemic in America. The reality is that HIV/AIDS in America acutely affects poor blacks in the American South. Although there have been some shifts in thinking in recent years, the general perception of AIDS in the United States is that it is a disease of white gay men in New York and San Francisco. This way of viewing AIDS often competes with the "global AIDS" story, which focuses on AIDS in Africa, but neither view does much to address the real and growing problem of AIDS in the United States. Any history of HIV in America that gives short-shrift to AIDS in minority communities or southern states is telling only half the story. Expanding the vision of what constitutes the AIDS story in the United States is particularly important because local and federal distribution of funding has relied on certain versions of that story. As Richard Rumley found out, there was no AIDS in eastern North Carolina until he and his team pointed it out. Likewise, the Southern AIDS Coalition has shown ways that federal formulas underestimate the scope of AIDS in the American South, despite the clear and growing burden AIDS places on southern health infrastructures. Broadening the AIDS story has more than historiographical value.

One of the most important themes of the story of AIDS in North Carolina is that southern states were able to contain the epidemic in white gay communities but proved unable to curb its spread in African American communities. As I have argued, simplistic claims of racism, classism, homophobia, or conservative opposition will not do; a host of factors brought about this state of affairs. AIDS, as Richard Rumley would argue, was in many ways a symptom of a much more deep-seated set of problems in American society. Some of the most important factors were historical and structural, and they will continue to determine the health of minority communities long after clinicians find a cure for HIV infection. Some of the factors relate to American values: Americans on both the Right and the Left tend both to stress individual autonomy at the expense of community well-being and to search for singular rather than polyphonic solutions to problems.[15] Any solution to the problem of HIV in America that privileges individual behavior issues over the social determinants of health will fail. Addressing the factors that drive an epidemic and that render certain populations more vulnerable to infection and transmission than others, is essential to eradicating HIV/AIDS in this country.

An additional issue this study brings to the fore is the problem of contextualization.[16] Recently, a great deal of attention has been paid to the "politics of difference in medical research," as researchers and activists have called for greater diversity in clinical research. Equally important, as this study points out, is the need to diversify the evidence base of public health interventions. One of the most profound struggles that AIDS educators encountered in North Carolina was reaching minority MSM, particularly those in rural communities or those who did not self-identify as gay. Groups like the LGHP tried unsuccessfully to translate programs that had worked among urban white gays to semi-urban black MSM, but they had no other evidence-based interventions to offer in their place. When the entire infrastructure of AIDS exceptionalism depends on inciting voluntary testing and behavior change through community awareness, what is one left with when outreach efforts consistently fail? For years, North Carolina had no answer to that question, and the ongoing resistance to implementing routine opt-out testing across North Carolina and the United States only ensures that these "missed opportunities" for early detection and treatment will persist. Understanding the short- and long-term consequences of public health interventions—as well as seemingly unrelated policy issues like incarceration policy—is an essential component to comprehending the epidemic in the United States.[17]

I can imagine a follow-up question to the one posed by my students at the beginning of this book: What will it take to solve the problem of AIDS in black communities? I would tell them that the answer lies in community and I would read to them a passage from an article Richard Rumley wrote in 1994:

> I believe that the secret to stopping AIDS, teenage pregnancies, domestic violence and drugs will not be discovered in a modern laboratory, developed in a leading hospital, decided in a court of law, or written in the legislative chambers. These problems can be solved when we see that these problems are actually the late terminal symptoms of a "futureless future." We as a society on the streets of our communities must prevent [any] child's existence from being despised. . . . We cannot legislate a future with opportunity and promise; it's going to take people helping people. We need to buy into this despair, carry some of it with us, invest in it, if we are to help children see and feel their true worth. If they work hard, go to school, get a job, everything's going to be okay, that's a lie. We've got to show them the way to opportunity, equip them with the skills and tools to dig their way out of a futureless future. Each one of us must embrace this responsibility because within it lies the true promise of a future.[18]

As the work of David Jolly, Howard Fitts, Evelyn Foust, Richard Rumley, and Louise Alston suggests, reducing HIV in our most vulnerable communities will require, in Friedrich Nietzsche words, "a long obedience in the same direction"; it will not come through a quick fix.[19] It will demand cooperation from government and individuals, families and organizations. And our efforts cannot merely aim to tackle the presenting disease without paying attention to, and doing something about, the underlying sociostructural determinants of health in our communities. This is true for HIV in North Carolina and the American South, and it is true for countless other diseases as well. Only then will we be able to offer our communities, both young and old, a future and a hope.

NOTES

Introduction

1. All quotes in the next two paragraphs, except where indicated, are from Spivey, "2." For more on North Carolina's STAT program, see North Carolina Department of Health and Human Services, Division of Public Health, HIV/STD Prevention and Care Branch, "Chapter 5: Special Studies," 65–66.

2. CDC, "HIV Transmission among Black College Student and Non-Student Men."

3. CDC, "HIV Transmission among Black Women."

4. Shilts, *And the Band Played On*; Kramer, *Reports from the Holocaust*; Kramer, *Normal Heart*; Kushner, *Angels in America*; Rene, *Longtime Companion*; Holleran, *Ground Zero*; Friedman and Joslin, *Silverlake Life*.

5. White and Cunningham, *Ryan White*; Kirp, *Learning by Heart*.

6. Bayer, *Private Acts, Social Consequences*. Other works, like Perrow and Guillen, *AIDS Disaster*, and Patton, *Inventing AIDS*, highlighted the unique nature of AIDS in the ways that elites framed the problem of AIDS to influence public policy, direct public health priorities, and gain personal power.

7. Bayer, "Clinical Progress," 1042.

8. Bayer and Edington, "HIV Testing, Human Rights, and Global AIDS Policy."

9. Stengel, Cronin, and Holmes, "Changing Face of AIDS," 13.

10. Bayer, *Private Acts, Social Consequences*, 4.

11. Hammonds, "Missing Persons"; Hammonds, "Seeing AIDS," 115; Juhasz, "Contained Threat." See also "AIDS: Its Impact on Women, Children, and Families."

12. King and Hunter, *On the Down Low*. For a thorough review of popular and scholarly perspectives on the "Down Low," see Ford et al., "Black Sexuality."

13. Oppenheimer, "In the Eye of the Storm"; Connor and Kingman, *Search for the Virus*; Gallo, *Virus Hunting*; Montagnier, *Virus*; Nussbaum, *Good Intentions*; Valdiserri, *Dawning Answers*; Jon Cohen, *Shots in the Dark*.

14. Epstein, *Impure Science*; Epstein, *Inclusion*; Kramer, *Reports from the Holocaust*; McGovern, "Barriers to the Inclusion of Women."

15. North Carolina Department of Health and Human Services, Division of Public Health, HIV/STD Prevention and Care Branch, *N.C. Epidemiologic Profile* (2005), 15. In 2004, the rate of HIV infection for non-Hispanic blacks was 58.9; and for non-Hispanic whites, 7.6. HIV infection among black non-Hispanic males was 84.0; and for white non-Hispanic males, 12.9. HIV infection among black non-Hispanic females was 36.4; and for white non-Hispanic females, 2.5.

16. According to the North Carolina Department of Health and Human Services,

Division of Public Health, HIV/STD Prevention and Care Branch, *N.C. Epidemiologic Profile* (2005), "In 2004, Hertford County had the highest county HIV infection rate (based on a 3-year average for 2002–2004) of 71.7 per 100,000 population. This was more than three times the state's three-year average rate of 21.7 per 100,000 population. Edgecombe County ranked second with an HIV rate of 55.2, followed by Mecklenburg County (48.8), Durham County (41.3), and Duplin County (36.6)" (15–16).

17. I am using the CDC's definition of the South here, which encompasses the following states: Alabama, Arkansas, Delaware, Florida, Georgia, Kentucky, Louisiana, Maryland, Mississippi, North Carolina, Oklahoma, South Carolina, Tennessee, Texas, Virginia, West Virginia, and the District of Columbia.

18. CDC, *HIV/AIDS Surveillance Report*, 2007.

19. Ibid.

20. Southern AIDS Coalition, *Southern States Manifesto*, 4; CDC, "Estimated Numbers of Adults and Adolescents Living with AIDS by Region, Slide 7."

21. CDC, *HIV/AIDS Surveillance Report*, 2007, 1–63. At the time those statistics were available, thirty-four states provided the CDC with long-term, confidential name–based HIV reporting.

22. CDC, "Proportions of AIDS Cases among Adults and Adolescents, Slide 2."

23. CDC, *HIV/AIDS Surveillance Report*, 2007.

24. Gilman, *Disease and Representation*, 4.

25. See, for example, Cathy J. Cohen, *Boundaries of Blackness*; and Hammonds, "Seeing AIDS."

26. Southern State AIDS Directors Work Group, *Southern States Manifesto*, 14.

27. Mackenzie, "Scientific Silence."

28. Verghese, *My Own Country*.

29. Whetten-Goldstein and Nguyen, *"You're the First One I've Told."*

30. Cathy J. Cohen, *Boundaries of Blackness*.

31. Levenson, *Secret Epidemic*.

32. Ibid., 275.

33. Wallace, "Synergism of Plagues"; Adimora et al., "Concurrent Sexual Partnerships among African Americans"; Aral, Adimora, and Fenton, "Understanding and Responding to Disparities in HIV"; Thomas, "From Slavery to Incarceration."

34. Luloff, Miller, and Beaulieu, "Social Conservatism"; Chen and Lind, "Political Economy of Beliefs"; Lichtenstein, Hook, and Sharma, "Public Tolerance, Private Pain."

35. For some insight into the complex and variegated nature of social conservatives, see Schoenwald, *Time for Choosing*; Christian Smith, *Christian America?*; and Zimmerman, *Whose America?*

Chapter 1

1. Pressley, ". . . Another's Frightening Future."

2. In 1970, in a basement building along Chapel Hill's Franklin Street, he opened one of the area's first gay bars, the Pegasus.

3. On Rowand's sexual history, see Pressley, ". . . Another's Frightening Future." Amyl and butyl nitrates are liquid chemical mixtures that reduce the blood pressure and accelerate the heart rate, thereby relaxing the involuntary muscles (especially the blood vessel walls and the anal sphincter). Among partners engaging in anal sex, they serve the dual purpose of heightening sexual arousal and relaxing the anus for penetration. Early epidemiological theories about AIDS centered on butyl nitrates as a factor in immune suppression. See Poulsen, "Alkyl Nitrite as an Aphrodisiac"; and Jaffe et al., "National Case-Control Study of Kaposi's Sarcoma."

4. The term "frightening future" comes from Pressley, ". . . Another's Frightening Future."

5. Associated Press, "AIDS-Patient Confidentiality"; "Carolinas Cases"; Smiley interview.

6. "Carolinas Cases"; Pressley, "One Victim's Final, Horrible Days."

7. "North Carolina AIDS Cases Diagnosed between pre-1982 and 1983," in CDC, AIDS Public Information Data Set (hereafter APIDS). See also "Carolinas Cases."

8. Department of Geography and Earth Sciences, University of North Carolina at Charlotte, North Carolina Atlas Revised.

9. Ibid.

10. Arrington, "IV-Drug Use Injects Durham"; Drug Enforcement Administration, *Drug Enforcement Administration*, 59–61; Dombey-Moore, Resetar, and Childress, *System Description of the Cocaine Trade*, cited in Cook et al., "What's Driving an Epidemic?"

11. Rumley interview.

12. David Jolly, "North Carolina Lesbian and Gay Health Survey: Summary Report, 1983–1985, June 1985," 1–27, Box 8, The Programming and Services Series, North Carolina Lesbian and Gay Health Project Records, Rare Book, Manuscript, and Special Collections Library, Duke University, Durham (hereafter LGHP Records). Truckers and truck stops also played a role in the spread of HIV/AIDS in the Southeast; see Verghese, *My Own Country*, 115–16, 135–36.

13. Smith and Gentry, "Migrant Farm Workers' Perceptions"; Associated Press, "Migrants' Poor Health Blamed on Isolation"; McClain, "Migrant Workers Travel a Hard Road"; "Epidemiologic Notes and Reports: HIV Seroprevalence"; Associated Press, "Study Indicates N.C. Migrant Workers Have High Rate of AIDS Infection"; "AIDS and Migrant Workers."

14. "Carolinas Cases"; Smiley interview.

15. Contaminated blood and blood products also served as a means of HIV transmission into the state. See CDC, "Epidemiologic Notes and Reports *Pneumocystis Carinii* Pneumonia among Persons with Hemophilia A"; Allen and Koepke, "Look Back"; Verghese, *My Own Country*, 232; and Shepard, "Experts Weigh AIDS Risk."

16. CDC, "1992 National Health Interview Survey"; "Bad News Is Getting Worse"; Thomas and Quinn, "Tuskegee Syphilis Study." See also James H. Jones, *Bad Blood*; and Katz, "Scientists Link Stress, Hypertension in Blacks."

17. Darrow, "Venereal Infections"; Irwin et al. "Sexually Transmitted Disease Patients' Self-Treatment Practices," 301.

18. Farley, "Sexually Transmitted Diseases." See also W. J. Wilson, *When Work Disappears*; and W. J. Wilson, *Truly Disadvantaged*.

19. Myron S. Cohen, "HIV and Sexually Transmitted Diseases." Cohen notes that "Sexually transmitted diseases (STDs) can increase risk for acquisition and transmission of HIV via a number of mechanisms, including breaching of mechanical barriers to infection, increased inflammation and higher levels of HIV cellular targets, and increased genital tract HIV levels" (104). For other research on the "lethal synergy" of concomitant STIs, see Piot, "AIDS"; Wasserheit, "Epidemiological Synergy"; and Advisory Committee for HIV and STD Prevention, "HIV Prevention."

20. Division of STD Prevention, *Sexually Transmitted Disease Surveillance*, 2002; David Jolly, "North Carolina Lesbian and Gay Health Survey: Summary Report, 1983–1985, June 1985," 1–27, LGHP Records.

21. Adimora and Schoenbach, "Social Context"; Kretzschmar and Morris, "Measures of Concurrency."

22. On gay men, see Jolly, "North Carolina Lesbian and Gay Health Survey: Summary Report, 1983–1985, June 1985," 20, LGHP Records. On minorities, see Adimora et al., "Concurrent Sexual Partnerships among Women"; and Adimora et al., "Concurrent Sexual Partnerships among African Americans."

23. See Laumann and Youm, "Racial/Ethnic Group Differences."

24. APIDS, 2002.

25. See, for example, Hopkins, "Inspired to Dance"; and Sullivan, "Bibliographic Guide to Government Hearings and Reports." Between 1977 and 1983, several gay-related hate crimes occurred, including the Raleigh "police riot" against a gay block party in May 1977; the murder of an elderly gay man in Winston-Salem in October 1980; the killing of an Alamance County woman thought to be a lesbian by her estranged husband in 1981; and the murder of a gay department store executive in 1983. For a more detailed list of assorted gay-related hate crimes in North Carolina, see *Legal Guide*; and Ackerman et al., "Triangle Lesbian, Gay, Bisexual, and Transgender Community." See also *State v. Richardson*.

26. This data summarized from Ackerman et al., "Triangle Lesbian, Gay, Bisexual, and Transgender Community."

27. Lekus, "Health Care"; David Jolly, "The Lesbian and Gay Health Project of North Carolina: 1984: A Report to the Community, March 1985," Box 1, Administrative Series, Annual Reports, 1984–92/93, LGHP Records; LGHP, "Lesbian and Gay Health Project," 1983, Box 2, General Historical Information and Pamphlets, 1983–95, LGHP Records.

28. For more on this, see Buechler, *Social Movements in Advanced Capitalism*.

29. Jolly interview, November 8, 2007.

30. LGHP, "Lesbian and Gay Health Project, Spring 1983," Box 2, General Historical Information and Pamphlets, 1983–95, n.d., LGHP Records.

31. Ibid.

32. Ibid.

33. On Carl Wittman's important career in the New Left movements of the 1960s, see Schewel, "Carl Wittman"; and "Carl Wittman." Some observers maintain that

Wittman's impassioned 1970 essay "Refugees from Amerika: A Gay Manifesto" helped ignite the West Coast's gay liberation movement. See Wittman, *Refugees from Amerika*; and Bronski, "Carnival as Organizing."

34. LGHP, "Lesbian and Gay Health Project, Spring 1983," Box 2, General Historical Information and Pamphlets, 1983–95, n.d., LGHP Records.

35. Ibid.

36. Ibid.; Jolly interviews, 2007; Adinolfi interview.

37. Jolly interview, November 8, 2007.

38. LGHP, "Lesbian and Gay Health Project, Spring 1983," Box 2, General Historical Information and Pamphlets, 1983–95, n.d., LGHP Records.

39. Jolly, "About the Lesbian/Gay Health Project." For more on this kind of response to the disease in various communities, see Valdiserri, "HIV/AIDS' Contribution to Community Mobilization."

40. On AIDS activists within the American organizing tradition, see Valdiserri, "HIV/AIDS in Historical Profile." On AIDS activism as an "American" response to AIDS, see Altman, *AIDS in the Mind of America*.

41. CDC, "Epidemiologic Notes and Reports *Pneumocystis Carinii* Pneumonia among Persons with Hemophilia A."

42. Associated Press, "Six Received Blood Product"; Shepard, "Experts Weigh AIDS Risk."

43. Weinberg et al., "Legal, Financial, and Public Health Consequences"; Keshavjee, Weiser, and Kleinman, "Medicine Betrayed"; Evatt, "Infectious Disease in the Blood Supply."

44. On the CDC's first transfusion report, see CDC, "Possible Transfusion-Associated Acquired Immunodeficiency Syndrome." On the institution of antibody screening in spring 1985, see Bayer, *Private Acts, Social Consequences*. On some of the earliest cases in North Carolina, see Allen and Koepke, "Look Back."

45. The quotes come from Jaffe, "Looking for a Common Thread." On AIDS numbers in North Carolina and the United States, see APIDS. On the inability of substance users to organize around AIDS, see Bayer and Kirp, "United States."

46. "Carolinas Cases."

47. Cathy J. Cohen, *Boundaries of Blackness*.

48. Jolly interview, December 21, 2007; Cathy J. Cohen, *Boundaries of Blackness*; Herdon interview, 2006; Bayer and Kirp, "United States."

49. Jolly interview, November 8, 2007.

50. Shilts, *And the Band Played On*, 325–27; National Lesbian and Gay Health Association Records, Division of Rare and Manuscript Collections, Cornell University Library, Ithaca, N.Y.

51. Shilts, *And the Band Played On*.

52. Ibid., 327.

53. Bayer and Kirp, "United States"; Valdiserri, "HIV/AIDS in Historical Profile," 3–30; Steffen, "Normalisation of AIDS Policies in Europe."

54. Jolly interview, November 8, 2007.

55. Pressley, ". . . Another's Frightening Future," 1, 11; Adinolfi interview.

56. The group included David Jolly, Carl Wittman, Timmer McBride, Sue Avery, Tony Adinolfi, Allen Troxler, Glenn Rowand, and Douglas Ruhren. See Jolly interview, November 8, 2007; Adinolfi interview, 2007; and Hamilton interview.

57. Duke had already gained national recognition on its work with AIDS growing out of the work of their chief of infectious diseases, Dr. David Durack. This was 1983, of course, about two years before an HIV antibody test became available. Thus most of these "worried well" went in to find out whether they had AIDS, pre-AIDS/ARC, or nothing discernable at all. "Most of the patients," Durack noted, did "not have symptoms . . . but just needed reassurance." While almost fifty had gone to visit the clinic, only twelve actually had the symptoms then associated with AIDS. See Connie Ballard, "AIDS: New Duke Clinic."

58. Ibid.

59. Ibid.

60. Earliest, in this case, means cases diagnosed prior to 1984. See APIDS. Many of the earliest cases among African Americans in North Carolina were diagnosed before 1984 but not reported until later.

61. Division of STD Prevention, *Sexually Transmitted Disease Surveillance*, 2002; Myron S. Cohen, "HIV and Sexually Transmitted Diseases." Cohen notes, "Sexually transmitted diseases (STDs) can increase risk for acquisition and transmission of HIV via a number of mechanisms, including breaching of mechanical barriers to infection, increased inflammation and higher levels of HIV cellular targets, and increased genital tract HIV levels" (Cohen, 2004, 104) For other research on the "lethal synergy" of concomitant STIs, see Piot, "AIDS"; Wasserheit, "Epidemiological Synergy"; and Advisory Committee for HIV and STD Prevention, "HIV Prevention."

62. Herndon interview, February 8, 2006. Racially segregated sexual networks are a national phenomenon in the United States; they are not limited to North Carolina. See Laumann and Youm, "Racial/Ethnic Group Differences." Since Asians, Hispanics, and American Indians only constituted a small portion of North Carolina's population in the 1980s, I have largely omitted them from this analysis.

63. See Laumann and Youm, "Racial/Ethnic Group Differences."

64. Guttentag and Secord, *Too Many Women*; Adimora and Schoenbach, "Social Context," 117–18.

65. "1990 Census of Population and Housing, North Carolina."

66. Thomas and Thomas, "Things Ain't What They Ought to Be."

67. Adimora and Schoenbach, "Social Context."

68. Adimora et al., "Concurrent Sexual Partnerships among Women"; Adimora et al., "Concurrent Sexual Partnerships among African Americans."

69. North Carolina's African American communities had participated in the post–Civil War farming economy until consolidation and mechanization drove agricultural workers—both black and white—from the land. As the American economy transformed into a service economy, implicit and explicit white supremacy in the state relegated African Americans—particularly African American men—to low-skilled, blue collar jobs or consigned them to long-term unemployment. See Davidson, *Broken Heartland*; Jong Mo Rhee, "Redistribution of the Black Work Force"; Farley,

"Sexually Transmitted Diseases"; Sugrue, *Origins of the Urban Crisis*; Hale, "'For Colored' and 'For White'"; Simon, "Race Reactions"; Nielsen and Alderson, "Income Inequality, Development, and Dualism"; Thomas and Thomas, "Things Ain't What They Ought to Be"; Massey, "American Apartheid"; Harrison and Weinberg, "How Important Were Changes"; and David Barton Smith, *Health Care Divided*.

70. "Civilian Labor Force Estimates."

71. Hossfeld, "Poverty in the East."

72. Farley, "Sexually Transmitted Diseases." See also W. J. Wilson, *When Work Disappears*; and W. J. Wilson, *Truly Disadvantaged*.

73. Department of Geography and Earth Sciences, University of North Carolina at Charlotte, North Carolina Atlas Revisted.

74. Ibid.

75. Braithwaite, "Irony of State Intervention," 142.

76. Rose and Clear, "Incarceration, Social Capital and Crime," 441; Braithwaite, "Irony of State Intervention."

77. Gorbach et al., "'It Takes a Village.'"

78. Cohen et al., "Potential Role of Custody Facilities."

79. CDC, "1992 National Health Interview Survey"; "Bad News Is Getting Worse."

80. Thomas and Quinn, "Tuskegee Syphilis Study." See also James H. Jones, *Bad Blood*; Katz, "Scientists Link Stress, Hypertension in Blacks."

81. Darrow, "Venereal Infections in Three Ethnic Groups"; Irwin, Thomas, Leone et al. "Sexually Transmitted Disease Patients' Self-Treatment," 301.

82. Stillwaggon, *AIDS and the Ecology of Poverty*, 45. For the most succinct summary of the ways co-morbidities promote infectious disease in general and HIV transmission in particular, see ibid., 31–66.

83. Valdiserri, "HIV/AIDS in Historical Profile"; Bayer and Kirp, "United States."

84. Valdiserri, "HIV/AIDS' Contribution to Community Mobilization"; Bayer and Kirp, "United States"; Noto interview, November 1, 2007; Jolly interview, November 8, 2007.

85. Bayer and Kirp, "United States."

86. Jolly interview, November 8, 2007. See also Bayer and Kirp, "United States."

87. Bayer and Kirp, "United States."

Chapter 2

1. This rendering of the story comes from facts gleaned from "Health Project Helps and Needs Help," and from a compilation of other stories of people with AIDS in the South.

2. Ibid.

3. Oral history interview by Cecil Wooten, Southern Oral History Program Collection, University of North Carolina, Chapel Hill.

4. Jaffe, "AIDS."

5. Ibid.

6. Twenty-nine percent of the men surveyed reported three or more years of

monogamy, 24 percent reported three or more sexual partners per month in the previous year, and 39 percent reported more than one hundred lifetime sexual partners. Additionally, 33 percent reported between one and six anonymous sexual contacts, and 39 percent reported seven or more. This level of sexual activity was comparable to that of a 1977 North American sample of gay men. See David Jolly, "The North Carolina Lesbian and Gay Health Survey: Summary Report, June 1985," Box 8, The Programming and Services Series, Surveys, North Carolina Lesbian and Gay Health Project Records, Rare Book, Manuscript, and Special Collections Library, Duke University, Durham (hereafter LGHP Records).

7. Leo Teachout, "Carl Wittman Letter, July 13, 1983," Box 2, Correspondence, 1983–84, LGHP Records; Mullis, "Health Project Update."

8. See, for example, Jolly, "About the Lesbian/Gay Health Project"; "AIDS Fight Deserves Support"; Jolly, "To the Readers of The FrontPage."

9. Carl Wittman focused more on awareness than "services" (Jolly interview, December 21, 2007).

10. Adinolfi interview.

11. Durack, "Opportunistic Infections."

12. Durack opened the clinic with fellow infectious disease specialist John Hamilton. See Russell, "Immunity Systems"; Ballard, "AIDS"; and Hamilton interview. AIDS patients came to Duke from as far away as the Caribbean; see Adinolfi interview.

13. "Carolinas Cases," 10; van der Horst interview, December 3, 2007. Pathologist Harold Roberts led the hemophilia center. See Associated Press, "Six Received Blood Product"; and "Roberts Honored by Dominican Republic President."

14. Adinolfi interview.

15. Ibid.

16. Ibid.

17. Shilts, *And the Band Played On*, 123, 188.

18. Jolly interview, December 21, 2007; Adinolfi interview; "Health Project Helps and Needs Help."

19. Jolly interview, December 21, 2007.

20. Adinolfi interview.

21. See Edward Brandt, "Concern about the Transmission of Acquired Immune Deficiency Syndrome: Letter to the Secretary of Health and Human Services," U.S. Department of Health and Human Services, June 22, 1983, Box 11, LGHP Records; Oleske et al. "Immune Deficiency Syndrome in Children"; and Fauci, "Acquired Immune Deficiency Syndrome."

22. See Smiley interview and van der Horst interview, 2007.

23. Jolly interview, December 21, 2007.

24. Adinolfi interview.

25. Ibid.

26. Ibid.

27. Smiley interview.

28. "Health Project Helps and Needs Help."

29. Ibid.

30. Ibid.

31. CDC, AIDS Public Information Data Set (hereafter APIDS).

32. "Health Project Helps and Needs Help."

33. See for example, Leo Teachout, "Health Survey Inquiry Letter," Box 2, Correspondence, 1983–84, LGHP Records. Jolly addressed AIDS at the Lesbian and Gay Health Conferences in Raleigh and Atlanta. See David Jolly, "The Lesbian and Gay Health Project of North Carolina: 1984: A Report to the Community, March 1985," Box 1, Administrative Series, Annual Reports, 1984–92/93, LGHP Records.

34. David Jolly, "The Lesbian and Gay Health Project of North Carolina: 1984: A Report to the Community, March 1985," Box 1, Administrative Series, Annual Reports, 1984–92/93, LGHP Records.

35. Adinolfi interview

36. N.C. Department of Health and Human Services, "North Carolina HIV Cases."

37. Herndon interview, 2006.

38. "AIDS Support Network—June 10, 1984," Box 11, Steering Committee Packets, 1983–84, LGHP Records.

39. "Carolinas Cases."

40. NGTF AIDS Program, "AIDS Advisory: Applying for Social Security Benefits —the Basic Fact, December 1983," Box 11, Subject Files Series, 1986–95, n.d., HIV/AIDS—Life Insurance, LGHP Records; Dante Noto, "Notes on Support Services, January 16, 1986," Box 1, Steering Committee Packets, 1986, LGHP Records.

41. Associated Press, "Division Seeks Reporting Rule"; "North Carolina Doctors to Report AIDS"; Levine interview. By this time, "at least 18 states and territories [had] made AIDS reportable, and approximately 26 [had] introduced or [were] considering measures to make it reportable" (CDC, "Current Trends Update," 389–91).

42. Pressley, "One Victim's."

43. Jolly interview, November 8, 2007.

44. David Jolly, "The Lesbian and Gay Health Project of North Carolina: 1984: A Report to the Community, March 1985," 4–5, Box 1, Administrative Series, Annual Reports, 1984–92/93, LGHP Records.

45. Levine interview.

46. Noto interview, 2007.

47. Ibid.

48. "Health Project Helps and Needs Help."

49. Noto interview, 2007.

50. Adinolfi interview.

51. Noto interview, 2007; David Jolly, "The Lesbian and Gay Health Project of North Carolina: 1984: A Report to the Community, March 1985," Box 1, Administrative Series, Annual Reports, 1984–92/93, LGHP Records.

52. Noto interview, 2007.

53. Ibid.

54. Ibid.

55. Adinolfi interview. See also "AIDS Support Network—June 10, 1984," Box 11, Steering Committee Packets, 1983–84, LGHP Records.

56. Jolly interview, November 8, 2007.

57. Leo Teachout, "Letter to Carl Wittman," Box 2, Correspondence, 1983–84, LGHP Records.

58. Jolly, "Bobby Reynolds Letter," Box 2, Correspondence, 1983–84, LGHP Records.

59. Ibid.

60. Trew, "AIDS." Later evidence shows the hospital forced him onto medical leave and stopped paying him one month later. See also Alvarado, "Easing Public's Fear"; Pear, "U.S. Files First AIDS Discrimination Charge"; and "US Finds Discrimination in Firing of AIDS Victim."

61. Trew, "AIDS."

62. Jolly interviews.

63. See Joint Meeting of North Carolina Gay and Lesbian Health Projects, "'Minutes,' April 26, 1986," Box 10, Community Connections Series, LGHP Records. See also "AIDS Task Force/AWARE History," 1986, LGHP Records; and Dante Noto and Tony Adinolfi, "AIDS Support Services, February 20, 1986," Box 1, Steering Committee Packets, 1986, LGHP Records.

64. Smiley interview.

65. Ibid.

66. Ibid.

67. Alvarado, "Durham Victim."

68. Smiley interview.

69. Barré-Sinoussi et al., "Isolation of a T-Lymphotropic Retrovirus"; Popovic et al., "Detection, Isolation, and Continuous Production of Cytopathic Retroviruses."

70. LGHP, "HIV Testing Recommendations," Box 5, The Programming and Services Series, 1983–95—HIV testing: Miscellaneous, 1985, n.d., LGHP Records; see also Bayer, "AIDS and the Making of an Ethics of Public Health."

71. David Jolly, "The Lesbian and Gay Health Project of North Carolina: 1984: A Report to the Community, March 1985," Box 1, Administrative Series, Annual Reports, 1984–92/93, LGHP Records.

72. LGHP, "The Lesbian and Gay Health Project, Spring 1983," Box 2, General Historical Information and Pamphlets, 1983–95, n.d., LGHP Records.

73. Adinolfi interview; Noto interview, 2007.

74. Spohn, "Officials Want AIDS Test"; LGHP, "HIV Testing Recommendations," Box 5, The Programming and Services Series, 1983–95—HIV testing: Miscellaneous, 1985, n.d., LGHP Records. See also Jolly interview, November 8, 2007, and Jolly, "HTLV-III: To Test or Not to Test?"

75. Steffen, "Normalisation of AIDS Policies in Europe."

76. Bayer and Kirp, "United States."

77. "AIDS News Update"; United Press International, "Falwell Urging Action";

Frame, "Church's Response to AIDS"; "Churches and AIDS"; "Editorial." For reports that implicate homosexuals and intravenous drug users as culpable in their AIDS infection, see Snow, "Opinion of the Times"; and Chambers, "Let's Talk."

78. Fauci, "Acquired Immune Deficiency Syndrome"; Rosenbrock et al., "Normalization of AIDS in Western European Countries"; Bayer and Kirp, "United States." On food handler concerns, see "Editorial." On fears about family contagion, see "Editorial" and van der Horst interview, 2007. For blood industry concerns, see Spohn, "Officials Want AIDS Test."

79. Steffen, "Normalisation of AIDS Policies in Europe"; Bayer and Kirp, "United States"; Valdiserri, "HIV/AIDS in Historical Profile."

80. Trew, "AIDS."

81. Bayer, "AIDS and the Making of an Ethics of Public Health."

82. Bayer and Kirp, "United States"; Bayer, "AIDS and the Making of an Ethics of Public Health"; Valdiserri, "HIV/AIDS' Contribution to Community Mobilization."

83. Jolly interview, December 21, 2007.

84. Jolly interview, November 8, 2007.

85. Jolly interview, December 21, 2007. On concerns over gay social integration and sexual privacy, see Bayer and Kirp, "United States"; Bayer, "AIDS and the Making of an Ethics of Public Health"; and Shilts, *And the Band Played On.*

86. Bayer and Kirp, "United States."

87. The LGHP records show that Jolly and Adinolfi had at least two meetings with Meriwether and her Health Department staff. The first, in February, came before the Food and Drug Administration had released the antibody test. At this meeting, Jolly and Adinolfi met with Meriwether, Frank Barnes, and Jim Fowler of the North Carolina Health Department's Communicable Disease Control Branch, and they also addressed a crowd of about two hundred Health Department staff. See "LGHP Outreaches: LGHP and Its Stand on HTLV-III Screening, February 11, 1985," Box 7, Presentations—Reports, 1985, LGHP Records. The follow-up meeting came on March 20, just weeks before the anonymous testing rollout. At this latter meeting, Meriwether, Fowler, Barnes, and three other STD educators met with Jolly and Adinolfi to discuss how the Health Department staff could collaborate with the gay community on testing and prevention programs. See "LGHP Technical Assistance, March 20, 1985," Box 7, Presentation—Reports, 1985, LGHP Records; and Jolly interview, December 21, 2007.

88. "LGHP Technical Assistance, March 20, 1985," Box 7, Presentation—Reports, 1985, LGHP Records; Jolly interview, December 21, 2007.

89. Levine interview.

90. Ibid.

91. Jolly interview, November 8, 2007.

92. Spohn, "Officials Want AIDS Test to Be Separate"; Simpson, "Wake to Offer Tests to Protect Blood Supply"; Levine interview.

93. On testing in New York City, see Bayer and Kirp, "United States." On HIV testing in North Carolina, see Levine interview and Jolly interview, December 21, 2007.

94. Simpson, "Wake to Offer Tests to Protect Blood Supply." The federal government provided grants equaling $180,000 over budget years 1986 and 1987 to fund the AIDS labs. In 1987 the state also secured $115,205 to help hospitals and health departments report AIDS cases. The state government added a total of $80,000 over these two years to supplement the system. See Rowe and Ryan, "Comparing State-Only Expenditures for AIDS," 424–29. See also Toler, "AIDS Battle."

95. Spohn, "Officials Want AIDS Test to Be Separate."

96. Ibid.

97. Ibid.

98. Buse, Mays, and Walt, *Making Health Policy*, 6.

99. Ibid.

100. Where physicians recorded race. Cf. APIDS.

101. For a detailed exploration of the racial aspects of HIV/AIDS reporting and prevention in the United States, see Cathy J. Cohen, *Boundaries of Blackness*, 78–148.

102. The statistics in this paragraph all come from APIDS.

103. Where physicians recorded race. Cf. APIDS.

104. Ibid.

105. Smiley interview. See also Valdiserri, "HIV/AIDS' Contribution to Community Mobilization."

Chapter 3

1. Alston interview.

2. Ibid.

3. Lee interview; Lipscomb interviews; Herndon interviews.

4. Herndon interview, 1994.

5. Lipscomb interview, 1994.

6. Ibid.

7. Ibid.

8. Alston interview.

9. Smiley interview.

10. Jolly interview, December 21, 2007.

11. Alvarado, "Doctors Urged."

12. Jolly interview, December 21, 2007

13. Smiley interview.

14. Jones interview.

15. Ibid.

16. Koop, "Surgeon General's Report"; Toler, "AIDS Battle"; "AIDS Education Question."

17. Martin, "Authority on AIDS Says Battle Raging in Public Opinion."

18. Associated Press, "AIDS Education Bill Filed in House."

19. The number of states requiring AIDS education in school curriculums tripled between the summer and winter of 1987. The sixteen states were Alabama, Delaware, Georgia, Hawaii, Illinois, Iowa, Kansas, Maryland, Nevada, New Mexico, New

York, Ohio, Oklahoma, Pennsylvania, Rhode Island, and Virginia, and the District of Columbia. For a blow-by-blow description of debates over the first AIDS curriculum in the state, see Associated Press, "Senate OKs Revised AIDS Education Bill"; Associated Press, "Martin: Aids Focus"; Associated Press, "AIDS Education Plan"; Associated Press, "States that Require AIDS Education"; Graves, "AIDS Curriculum"; Graves, "Board of Education OKs Revised AIDS Curriculum"; and Jolly interview, November 8, 2007.

20. Jolly interview, December 21, 2007; "AIDS Education Question"; Associated Press, "Prison Bills Might Avert Federal Action"; North Carolina Department of Health and Human Services, "State-Wide Community Conference on AIDS."

21. Vauaghan, "Hello, AIDS Hotline?"; Jolly, "AIDS: Information"; Associated Press, "Prison Bills Might Avert Federal Action."

22. Bayer, *Private Acts, Social Consequences.* For more on the various debates, see Vauaghan, "Hello, AIDS Hotline?"; Jolly, "AIDS: Information"; and Associated Press, "Prison Bills Might Avert Federal Action."

23. North Carolina was one of only nine states to include AIDS in its quarantine law in 1987. See Lewin, "Rights of Citizens." On the other legislative debates, see Pride and Mellnik, "N.C. Bill Would Deny Licenses"; Garloch, "N.C. Legislators Debating How to Attack AIDS"; Associated Press, "N.C. House Rejects Mandatory AIDS Tests"; Funk, "Chairmen Let Many Bills Die"; Taylor, "Legislator Criticizes Failure of AIDS Bills"; Associated Press, "N.C. House Accepts Senate's Version of Bill on AIDS"; Garloch, "Clause on Housing Cut from AIDS Bill"; and Associated Press, "Panel Backs Elections between Presidential Races."

24. CDC, "Current Trends: Partner Notification."

25. For more on AIDS exceptionalism, see Bayer, "Entering the Second Decade."

26. Associated Press, "N.C. Seeks Grant for AIDS Programs."

27. NC AIDS Program, *AIDS.*

28. Garloch, "Plan for Tackling AIDS under Attack."

29. Ibid.

30. Garloch, "N.C. AIDS Plan Apparently Unique."

31. Jones interview.

32. Jolly interview, December 21, 2007.

33. Associated Press, "Task Force Offers Final Proposal for AIDS Rules."

34. Funk, "N.C. Health Officials Hedge on AIDS Rule."

35. Garloch, "AIDS Project Keeps Step with Disease."

36. Ibid.

37. McClain and Garloch, "Chambers Insists County Pull AIDS Support Group's Money"; "Avoid Demagoguery on AIDS."

38. McClain and Garloch, "Chambers Insists County Pull AIDS Support Group's Money"; Pullen, "Autrey Reverses Stance."

39. Pullen, "Autrey Reverses Stance."

40. Garloch, "AIDS."

41. Jones interview.

42. ACRA, "AIDS Community Residence Task Force, Minutes: May 28, 1987," Box

10, ACRA (Durham), 1987–95, LGHP Records; ACRA, "AIDS Community Residence Task Force, June 1987," Box 10, ACRA (Durham), 1987–95, LGHP Records. See also Associated Press, "Group Seeks Donations for AIDS House."

43. Associated Press, "Group Seeks Donations for AIDS House."

44. "Folksinger's Tunes to Help Raise Funds for AIDS Houses."

45. Ibid; Associated Press, "Group Seeks Donations for AIDS House."

46. Chip Wilson, "Gaston Seeks Battle Plan against AIDS"; Mullen, "HIV Task Force"; Moss, "Epidemic Just Beginning to Be Felt"; Moss, "Faith in God Gave Solace from Fear"; Helms, "AIDS Council Faces More Cases."

47. Tescher, "Syphilis Cases Today?"; Colwell, "Tracey Marshall's Message Lives On"; Mitchell, "More People Learn About—and Turn to—AIDS Alliance"; Jim Jones, "AIDS Effort Under Way."

48. Rocco Patt, "Letter to Jill Duvall, June 26, 1987," W.N.C. AIDS Project, Box 2, Correspondence, 1987, North Carolina Lesbian and Gay Health Project Records, Rare Book, Manuscript, and Special Collections Library, Duke University, Durham (hereafter LGHP Records); "Bylaws of ERASE," Greenville, N.C.: Eastern Regional AIDS Support and Education, September 14, 1987, Box 10, ERASE, LGHP Records.

49. Garloch, "AIDS Fear Rivals Cancer, Heart Ills." A statewide survey in 1987 indicated that 63 percent of black respondents considered AIDS to be the community's largest health threat; 30 percent felt personally affected; and 31 percent had taken precautions.

50. Hart-Brothers interview; Fitts interview.

51. Fitts interview; Durham Committee Institute, "Proposal: Clearinghouse and Network Center."

52. Fitts interview.

53. Campbell, *Women, Families, & HIV/AIDS*, 5.

54. Herndon interview; Lipscomb interview, 2008; "The Pink Triangle, January, 1987," Box 10, LGHP Records; Cathy J. Cohen, *Boundaries of Blackness*, 149–249; Lekus, "Health Care"; Dalton, "AIDS in Blackface"; Peterson and Marin, "Issues in the Prevention of AIDS."

55. Jolly interview, December 21, 2007.

56. Peterson and Marin, "Issues in the Prevention of AIDS"; Cathy J. Cohen, *Boundaries of Blackness*, 99, 104; Lekus, "Health Care."

57. Rogers and Williams, "AIDS a Big Problem among Blacks, Hispanics"; Robertson, "AIDS Is Equal-Opportunity Killer"; Hey, "Education Emphasized"; Weatherford and Weatherford, *Somebody's Knocking at Your Door*; Soderberg, "Black Churches Urged to Join Fight on AIDS."

58. Alston interview.

59. Ibid.

60. Ibid.

61. Smiley interview.

62. Jolly interview, November 8, 2007.

63. The funds went to the Durham County Health Department, the Durham Committee Institute, the AIDS Services Project (Durham), Step One/AIDS Task Force

(Winston-Salem), the Western North Carolina AIDS Project, Metrolina AIDS Project (Mecklenburg County), AIDS Awareness in the Black Community (New Hanover County Health Department), Operation Sickle Cell (Cumberland County), Planned Parenthood (Orange County), Drug Action (Wake County), and the Wake County Health Department. See Jolly interview, December 21, 2007; Vanderbush personal communication; Garloch, "Kooyman Rejected for Panel," 1C; Jolly, "Extension of Deadline for AIDS Education Projects"; Jones interview; and Garloch, "AIDS Agency, Others Still Wait for N.C."

64. The minority-focused programs were 1) Durham Committee Institute, 2) AIDS Awareness in the Black Community on behalf of the New Hanover County Health Department, 3) Cumberland County's Operation Sickle Cell, 4) Planned Parenthood on behalf of the Orange County Health Department, and 5) a consortium headed by the Wake County Health Department. Some of the recipients had applied for funds for multiple programs, but the state tried to spread the money out. Metrolina AIDS Project (Mecklenburg County) submitted an $80,000 minority AIDS program proposal on top of their program targeting men who have sex with men, for example, but lost out to James Rapp's East Winston Project in Winston-Salem. See Garloch, "AIDS Agency, Others Still Wait for N.C."; Garloch, "County, AIDS Group Get $29,500 Grant"; and Rapp, "Innovative Projects Focusing on the Prevention of AIDS."

65. Durham Committee Institute, "Proposal: Clearinghouse and Network Center."

66. The counties were Caswell, Durham, Edgecombe, Granville, Halifax, Nash, Person, Vance, Warren, and Wilson. See Durham Committee Institute, "Clearinghouse and Network Center for AIDS Education."

67. Durham Committee Institute, "Clearinghouse and Network Center for AIDS Education"; Durham Committee Institute, "Clearinghouse and Network Center for AIDS Education, Quarterly Report."

68. On the development of the Cumberland County program, for example, see Cunningham, "10-County Region Reports 89 Cases of AIDS since 1984"; McKenzie, "Health Counselors Going to Church"; Youngblood, "AIDS Story Is Survival "; and Womble, "Taking It to the Streets."

69. Jolly interview, November 8, 2007.

70. Ibid.

71. CDC, AIDS Public Information Data Set.

72. John Fletcher, "Jill Duval, Project Straightalk Letter, July 11, 1990," Box 2, Reducing Our Risk—Administrative and Financial Papers, 1989–90, LGHP Records; Arrington, "IV-Drug Use Injects Durham."

73. Alston interview.

74. Ibid.

75. Alston interview; Rutherford interview.

76. Jolly interview, December 21, 2007.

77. Goldstein, "AIDS and Race."

Chapter 4

1. Lipscomb interview, 2008.

2. Ibid.

3. Jolly interview, December 21, 2007.

4. Womble, "AIDS Awareness."

5. Durham Committee Institute, "Clearinghouse and Network Center for AIDS Education, Quarterly Report."

6. Durham Committee Institute, "Proposal: Clearinghouse and Network Center."

7. Durham Committee Institute, "Clearinghouse and Network Center for AIDS Education, Quarterly Report."

8. Ibid.

9. Ibid

10. Paddock, "Project Would Give AIDS Victims Last Home," 1D.

11. Allegood, "AIDS."

12. The North Carolina Council of Churches, "Task Force on AIDS," in North Carolina Council of Churches Records, Rare Book, Manuscript, and Special Collections Library, Duke University, Durham, N.C.

13. Garloch, "AIDS Network Wins Grant"; Garloch, "Congregations Reach out in an AIDS Ministry."

14. Moore, "Alliance's Mission."

15. Wilkie, "Minorities Offered AIDS Education."

16. Brown, Smith, and Suchetka, "How Safe Is Sex?"; Morehouse, "Calls to AIDS Hotline Jump."

17. Mangle and Garloch, "AIDS Project Now Offers New Services"; McClain, "Candlelight Vigil Pays Tribute."

18. Morehouse, "7-County Region Gets Grant."

19. Ibid; Glendy, "People with AIDS Share Pain"; Helms, "Town Meeting on AIDS."

20. Jim Jones, "AIDS Effort Under Way."

21. Ibid.

22. Ibid.

23. Moose, "Women and AIDS."

24. Zepp, "Durham HIV Clinic to Expand Services."

25. The statistics for women and adolescents are based on data from North Carolina's three major metropolitan areas, and the data on children comes from statewide data in the CDC's AIDS Public Information Data Set (hereafter APIDS).

26. Some researchers have looked to biological explanations for the increased susceptibility of certain African Americans to HIV. See He et al., "Duffy Antigen Receptor for Chemokines." Other researchers have suggested more controversial explanation—the r-K theory of human evolution—maintaining that biological and histo-cultural differences between the races explain different rates of STIs and HIV/AIDS. See Rushton, *Race, Evolution, and Behavior*; and Lynn, "Race Differences in

Sexual Behavior." However, these conclusions seem profoundly problematic for what they ignore. See Farley "Sexually Transmitted Diseases."

27. Zaleski and Schiaffino, "Religiosity and Sexual Risk-Taking Behavior."

28. Farley, "Sexually Transmitted Diseases."

29. van der Horst interview, 1998.

30. CDC, "1992 National Health Interview Survey."

31. Irwin, Thomas, and Leone, "Sexually Transmitted Disease Patients' Self-Treatment Practices," 301.

32. Moss, "Brush with Death."

33. Ibid.

34. Alston interview.

35. Associated Press, "Workshop Focus."

36. "Bleak Future Seen for Poor with AIDS."

37. Jolly interview, November 8, 2007.

38. Fullilove et al. "Risk of Sexually Transmitted Disease."

39. Rengert, *Geography of Illegal Drugs*, cited in Cook et al., "What's Driving an Epidemic?"

40. Arrington, "Displaced Children Have No Place to Go"; Arrington, "IV-Drug use Injects Durham."

41. Arrington, "Displaced Children Have No Place to Go."

42. Rengert, *Geography of Illegal Drugs*.

43. Richissin, "This Corner Is the End of the Road."

44. Associated Press, "Gonorrhea, Syphilis on Rise in N.C."; Arrington, "Displaced Children Have No Place to Go."

45. Arrington, "IV-Drug Use Injects Durham."

46. Arrington, "Displaced Children Have No Place to Go"; Arrington, "IV-Drug Use Injects Durham."

47. Adimora et al., "Concurrent Partnerships among Rural African Americans"; Laumann and Youm, "Racial/Ethnic Group Differences."

48. Twenty-one percent of African Americans reported concurrent partnerships compared to 12 percent reported by the population as a whole, and sexual concurrency rates were as high as 60 percent in the mid-1990s in some rural black communities. See Adimora et al., "Concurrent Sexual Partnerships among African Americans"; and Adimora et al., "Concurrent Partnerships among Rural African Americans." According to the latter article, 38 percent of African Americans in North Carolina reported concurrent sexual partnerships in the previous five years. See also Morris and Kretzschmar, "Concurrent Partnerships"; Anderson, "Transmission Dynamics"; and Thomas, "From Slavery to Incarceration."

49. Laumann and Youm, "Racial/Ethnic Group Differences." Blacks were five times more likely than whites and four times more likely than Hispanics to have a sexual partner who had had multiple sexual partners. See Thomas and Thomas, "Things Ain't What They Ought to Be."

50. Governor's Crime Commission, "Crime and Justice in North Carolina"; U.S.

Department of Justice, Office of Justice Programs, Office of Juvenile Justice and Delinquency Prevention, "Evaluation of the Disproportionate Minority Confinement (DMC) Initiative."

51. Tonry, *Malign Neglect*, 113.

52. Wohl et al., "HIV Transmission Risk Behaviors."

53. Thomas and Torrone, "Incarceration as Forced Migration"; Clear et al., "Coercive Mobility and Crime."

54. Allegood, "AIDS."

55. "AIDS Cases Swamping N.C. Prisons."

56. Associated Press, "State Survey Focuses on AIDS Problem in Prison."

57. "AIDS Cases Swamping N.C. Prisons."

58. Ibid. The national average for state prisons was 2.8 percent.

59. Associated Press, "State Survey Focuses on AIDS Problem in Prison."

60. "AIDS Cases Swamping N.C. Prisons"; "Prisons Fear Start of AIDS Epidemic"; Boyce, "Prisons Seek Aid for AIDS."

61. Alston interview.

62. Fitts interview.

63. Frey, "New Great Migration"; Jong Mo Rhee, "Redistribution of the Black Work Force."

64. Frey, "New Great Migration"; Robinson, "Blacks Move Back to the South."

65. Adelman, Morett, and Tolnay, "Homeward Bound."

66. "1990 Census of Population and Housing, North Carolina."

67. Thomas and Gaffield, "Social Structure."

68. Ibid. See also Aral, "Social Context of Syphilis Persistence"; Tucker and Taylor, "Demographic Correlates of Relationship."

69. Smith and Gentry, "Migrant Farm Workers' Perceptions." See also Associated Press, "Migrants' Poor Health Blamed on Isolation"; and McClain, "Migrant Workers Travel a Hard Road."

70. "Epidemiologic Notes and Reports: HIV Seroprevalence"; "AIDS and Migrant Workers."

71. Associated Press, "Study Indicates N.C. Migrant Workers Have High Rate of AIDS Infection"; "AIDS and Migrant Workers"; Ciesielski et al., "Epidemiology of Tuberculosis"; Weber et al., "Epidemiology of Tuberculosis"; Califano, "Three-Headed Dog from Hell."

72. Rutherford interview.

73. Cathy Cohen discusses this in greater detail in her section on secondary marginalization in Cohen, *Boundaries of Blackness*, 70–76.

74. Rutherford interview.

75. Lipscomb interview, 1994; Rutherford interview.

76. Rutherford interview.

77. Lipscomb interview, 2008.

78. Rutherford interview.

79. Lipscomb interview, 2008.

80. Morehouse, "7-County Region Gets Grant."

81. Jim Jones, "AIDS Effort Under Way."

82. Adinolfi interview; Jill Duvall, "Old, New, and Present Steering Committee Members Letter, June 30, 1988," Box 1, Board of Directors—Membership and Correspondence, 1988–89, LGHP Records; Jill Duvall, "Welcome New Staff Members," North Carolina Lesbian and Gay Health Project Newsletter, December 1988, Box 1, Board of Directors—Membership and Correspondence, 1988–89, LGHP Records.

83. Jill Duvall, "Executive Director's Report, December 19, 1988," Box 1, Board Packets, 1988, LGHP Records.

84. Lavalle, "Internal Conflicts Challenge LGHP"; Noto interview, 1994; Lavalle, "Women in the AIDS Movement Face Criticism"; David Jones, "Jill Duvall Letter, March 18, 1989," Box 1, Board Packets, 1989, LGHP Records; Jill Duvall, "Executive Director's Report, December 19, 1988," Box 1, Board Packets, 1988, LGHP Records.

85. Lavalle, "Internal Conflicts Challenge LGHP"; David Jones, "Jill Duvall Letter, March 18, 1989," Box 1, Board Packets, 1989, LGHP Records; LGHP, "LGHP Board Minutes, March 20, 1989," Box 1, Board Packets, 1989, LGHP Records; LGHP, "Dear [Board member] Letter, April 12, 1989," Box 1, Board Packets, 1989, LGHP Records; LGHP, "LGHP Board Minutes, March 20, 1989," Box 1, Board Packets, 1989, LGHP Records; LGHP, "Minutes of the August, 1989 Meeting of Lesbian and Gay Health Project," Box 1, Board Packets, 1989, LGHP Records.

86. Adinolfi interview.

87. Jolly interview, November 8, 2007.

88. Jolly interview, December 21, 2007.

89. Adinolfi interview.

90. Duvall interview.

91. See LGHP, "LGHP Board Minutes, March 20, 1989," Box 1, Board Packets, 1989, LGHP Records; and Lavalle, "Internal Conflicts Challenge LGHP," 11.

92. Jones interview.

93. Tony Adinolfi, "Board of Directors Letter, July 19, 1989," Box 1, Board Packets, 1989, LGHP Records.

94. Noto interview, 1994.

95. Ibid.

96. Warden, "Activists Bemoan Scarcity of Blacks"; Jolly interview, November 8, 2007.

97. "NC AIDS Service Coalition Member Organizations," n.d., Box 1, Board Packets, 1989, LGHP Records.

98. Manuel, "Looming Crisis."

99. Warden, "Activists Bemoan Scarcity of Blacks."

100. Ibid.

101. Gladwell, "New Victims, Problems."

102. Lipscomb interview, 2008.

103. Ibid.

104. Baker and Elam, "Joining the AIDS Fight."

105. Durham Committee Institute, "AIDS Risk Reduction."

106. Alston interview; "Granville County AIDS Task Force Minutes, July 11, 1989," in Howard Fitts's personal collection; Durham Committee Institute, "Clearinghouse and Network Center for AIDS Education, Quarterly Report"; "Role of the Church in AIDS Education and Prevention."

107. Jolly, "Howard Fitts Letter, September 6, 1989."

108. Warden, "Activists Bemoan Scarcity of Blacks"; Jolly interview, November 8, 2007.

109. Warden, "Activists Bemoan Scarcity of Blacks"; Jolly interview, November 8, 2007.

110. Jolly interview, November 8, 2007.

111. Associated Press, "New Definition Triples Number."

112. Jolly interview, December 21, 2007. On the scarcity of African Americans in the public health education pipeline, see Crase and Walker, "Black Students and Professionals."

113. Associated Press, "New Definition Triples Number."

114. Jolly interview, December 21, 2007.

115. Ibid.

116. Jolly interview, November 8, 2007.

117. Ron Levine contends that they did this while he was out of the state. See Levine interview.

118. Jolly interview, December 21, 2007.

119. Ibid.; Jolly interview, November 8, 2007.

120. Jolly interview, December 21, 2007.

121. Associated Press, "N.C. Legislature Must Act."

122. Gutis, "Attacks on U.S. Homosexuals."

123. Garloch, "AIDS Needs Aren't Being Addressed."

124. "Children with AIDS Seen as No Threat"; Katherine White, "Most Children with AIDS Seen as No Threat"; "Martin: Policy Would Bar AIDS Discrimination"; Jones interview; Associated Press, "N.C. Legislature Must Act"; Associated Press, "Senate Oks AIDS Legislation."

125. Associated Press, "N.C. Legislature Must Act."

126. Associated Press, "AIDS Bill."

127. Associated Press, "N.C. Legislature Must Act"; Jones interview.

128. "AIDS Cases in N.C. Multiplying"; "AMA Says Tracing Could Fight AIDS"; Associated Press, "Senate Oks AIDS Legislation"; Jones interview.

129. Bayer, *Private Acts, Social Consequences.*

130. Jolly interview, December 21, 2007.

131. "AMA Says Tracing Could Fight AIDS"; "AIDS Warning Splits Doctors."

132. Stowe, "AIDS Test Anonymity in Question"; Garloch, "AIDS Report Focuses on Attitude"; Garloch, "AIDS Infighting"; Garloch, "Some MDs Push More AIDS Tests"; Associated Press, "Senate Oks AIDS Legislation."

133. "AMA Says Tracing Could Fight AIDS." For more on the impact zidovudine

and other AIDS therapies had on the public health push to end AIDS exceptionalism, see Bayer, *Private Acts, Social Consequences*

134. Van der Horst interview, 2007; Jones interview.

135. Jones interview; "Anonymous AIDS Tests Assured."

136. "Anonymous AIDS Testing on Agenda."

137. Ibid.

138. "Anonymous AIDS Tests Assured."

139. Jolly interview, November 8, 2007.

140. Ibid.

141. Ibid.

142. Ibid.

143. Jolly interview, December 21, 2007.

144. Jolly interview, November 8, 2007.

145. Ibid.

146. Levine interview.

147. Kanigel, "New Rule Could End AIDS Test Anonymity."

148. Catanoso, "Confidential AIDS Testing."

149. Kanigel, "New Rule Could End AIDS Test Anonymity."

150. Only eight states relied solely on named-based reporting. See Kanigel, "New Rule Could End AIDS Test Anonymity."

151. Levine interview.

152. Kanigel, "New Rule Could End AIDS Test Anonymity."

153. Ibid.

154. Williams, "AIDS Test Proposal Attacked."

155. Catanoso, "Confidential AIDS Testing."

156. Kanigel, "Continued Anonymity in AIDS Tests Urged."

157. Teachout, "Consider HIV Testing."

158. Paddock, "Save Lives."

159. Catanoso, "Confidential AIDS Testing."

160. Ibid.

161. "Doctor: Anonymous AIDS Test."

162. Jolly interview, November 8, 2007.

163. Ibid.

164. Ibid.

165. Williams, "AIDS Test Proposal Attacked."

166. Kanigel, "New Rule Could End AIDS Test Anonymity."

167. Kanigel, "State Places Limits on Anonymous Tests."

168. Bayer, *Private Acts, Social Consequences*, 72–136.

169. Kegeles et al., "Mandatory Reporting of HIV Testing"; Fordyce, Sambula, and Stoneburner, "Mandatory Reporting"; Kegeles et al., "Many People Who Seek Anonymous HIV-Antibody Testing."

170. For a detailed analysis of the literature, see Tesoriero et al., "Effect of Name-Based Reporting."

171. Levine interview; Kanigel, "State Places Limits on Anonymous Tests."

172. Kanigel, "State Places Limits on Anonymous Tests"; Kanigel, "Activists Seek Anonymous AIDS Testing."

173. Kanigel, "Activists Seek Anonymous AIDS Testing." On Lester Lee, see Jolly interview, November 8, 2007.

174. Hoar, "Request Denied."

175. Manuel, "Looming Crisis."

176. Warden, "Activists Bemoan Scarcity of Blacks."

177. Ibid. For more on the heavy social burdens facing many African American communities in the 1980s and 1990s, see Cathy J. Cohen, *Boundaries of Blackness*, 78–118.

178. Warden, "Activists Bemoan Scarcity of Blacks."

179. Gladwell, "New Victims, Problems."

180. Ibid.

181. Manuel, "Looming Crisis."

182. Ibid.

183. Warden, "Activists Bemoan Scarcity of Blacks."

184. Fitts interview.

185. Alston interview.

186. Baker and Elam, "Joining the AIDS Fight."

187. Ibid.

188. Manuel, "Looming Crisis."

189. Ibid.

190. Ibid.

191. Lipscomb interview, 2008

192. Manuel, "Looming Crisis."

193. Stephens, "United Way"; APIDS; Garloch, "N.C. Law Requires Doctors"; Garloch, "United AIDS Effort"; Manuel, "Looming Crisis."

194. Stephens, "United Way."

195. Ibid.

196. "AIDS Threat Growing among Women," A7; Garloch, "AIDS Virus Casts Deadly Shadow"; Stephens, "Adopting AIDS Child Proves Hard."

197. Moose, "Women and AIDS."

198. Ibid.

199. Ibid.; Maschal, "More Women Battle AIDS."

200. Moose, "Women and AIDS."

201. Alston interview.

202. Lipscomb interview, 2008.

203. Fitts interview.

204. Alston interview.

205. Fitts interview.

1. Quotes and content in the next two paragraphs taken from Maschal, "More Women Battle AIDS."

2. Gutis, "Attacks on U.S. Homosexuals"; "Martin: Policy Would Bar AIDS Discrimination"; Jones interview; Associated Press, "N.C. Legislature Must Act"; Associated Press, "Senate Oks AIDS Legislation."

3. Associated Press, "N.C. Legislature Must Act"; Jones interview.

4. Chandler, "High Cost of Failure."

5. Landis et al., "Results of a Randomized Trial."

6. Ibid.

7. Ibid.

8. Fulghum, "AIDS"; Halperin, "Informed Consent for AIDS Testing"; Bartlett, "HIV Testing in North Carolina."

9. Kanigel, "New Rule Could End AIDS Test Anonymity," A1.

10. Gauthier, "HIV Testing."

11. Fulghum, "AIDS."

12. CDC, AIDS Public Information Data Set (hereafter APIDS).

13. Fiscus et al., "Perinatal HIV Infection."

14. Arguably, however, improved surveillance could have reduced viral transmission via breast milk, so even here the surveillance restrictions seem misguided because restrictions neglected the nontherapeutic, public health value of surveillance.

15. Associated Press, "AIDS Case May Alter Transplant Policies."

16. Connor et al., "Reduction of Maternal-Infant Transmission."

17. Fiscus et al., "Perinatal HIV Infection"; Clabby, "State Testing Program."

18. Fiscus et al., "Perinatal HIV Infection."

19. Clabby, "State Testing Program." In 1996, federal legislators followed suit, requiring all states to have similar testing legislation (or the functional equivalent) in place by the year 2000.

20. Hood, "State House Sweep."

21. On the five of the thirty-seven fulfilled recommendations, see *Impact of AIDS in North Carolina.*

22. Primarily the bills HB 801 (the "HIV Assault" bill) and HB 834 (the "teach abstinence until marriage" bill).

23. General Assembly of North Carolina, 1995 Session, Chapter 534, House Bill 834.

24. Roslyn Savitt, *1995 North Carolina General Assembly Session, Legislative Report* (Raleigh: North Carolina HIV-AIDS Alliance, August 1995), Box 10, LGHP Records; "Schools Must Teach Abstinence."

25. Roslyn Savitt, *1995 North Carolina General Assembly Session, Legislative Report* (Raleigh: North Carolina HIV-AIDS Alliance, August 1995), Box 10, LGHP Records; "Schools Must Teach Abstinence."

26. Clemmons, "AIDS Outreach Called Frustrating"; Zimmer, "Board: Condoms Worth the Cost."

27. Carlson, "AIDS Home."

28. Jolly interview, December 21, 2007.

29. "Ryan White HIV Care Program, Summary, 1991," Box 6, PHHC, 1991–95 (folder 2 of 4), LGHP Records. By 1994, the state had 15 consortia covering 100 percent of the state with more than $1 million at its disposal. See "Ryan White Care Consortia in North Carolina, April 1, 1994," Box 6, PHHC, 1991–95 (folder 1 of 4), LGHP Records.

30. Bonnie Wilson, "Dogwood Consortium."

31. North Carolina AIDS Advisory Council, *NC/AIDS Index*.

32. Stan Holt, "Executive Director's Report, Jan. 13, 1993," Box 1, Board Packets, 1993, January–June, LGHP Records.

33. The AIDS Services Agency of Wake County, Inc., and LGHP, "Advocare Application, 1993," Box 1, The AIDS Service Project, Living Positively: Grants, Training Manuals, and Reports, 1992–94 (folder 2 of 2), LGHP Records. See also Cullen Gurganus, "Triangle Cooperative AIDS Task Force letter, September 24, 1993," Box 10, LGHP Records.

34. Jones interview.

35. McFadden, "Judge Overturns U.S. Rule"; "Finally Free to Speak Plainly?"; "Educators Denounce Brochure"; Wayne Bobbit Jr. "Stan Holt letter, May 14, 1993," North Carolina Department of Environment, Health, and Natural Resources, Unpublished letter, Box 7, Reducing Our Risk, Pamphlet Approval, 1991–93, LGHP Records.

36. See Stan Holt, "The AIDS Services Project, Reducing Our Risks Program, Monthly Report, February 1992," Box 1, Board Packets, 1992, January–June, LGHP Records; and Stan Holt, "The AIDS Services Project, Reducing Our Risks Program, Monthly Report, March 1992," Box 1, Board Packets, 1992, January–June, LGHP Records.

37. I am grateful to Stephen Thomas for his insight on some of these ideas about the organizational ecology of AIDS groups.

38. Zimmer, "Board: Condoms Worth the Cost."

39. In North Carolina, legislators originally set the criteria to qualify for medication assistance at an income 85 percent (or less) of the federal poverty level. See Zimmer, "AIDS Funding Evades State Budget Cuts." In 1995, the state legislature increased the eligibility level to 10 percent above the federal poverty level. By 1997, lawmakers had raised the amount to 25 percent above the federal poverty rate. See Kirkpatrick, "Cost of AIDS Drugs."

40. General Assembly of North Carolina, 1993 Session, Ratified Bill, Chapter 321, Senate Bill 27. See also General Assembly of North Carolina, 1993 Session, Senate Bill 695/House Bill 738. Prior to 1993, North Carolina was one of only eleven states that did not spend any of its own dollars on AIDS care. See Kirkpatrick, "Drugs Elusive for 22 Here."

41. Zimmer, "Housing Situation Often Tenuous."

42. This definition developed from Dombrowski, Thomas, and Kaufman, "Study in Contrasts."

43. Daniels, Kennedy, and Kawachi, "Justice Is Good for Our Health."

44. "Morbidity and Mortality Statistics," Table 5.

45. Porterfield, Dutton, and Gizlice, "Cervical Cancer in North Carolina."

46. "Pregnancy and Outcome Statistics," Table 4; Porterfield, Dutton, and Gizlice, "Cervical Cancer in North Carolina."

47. *1990 Census of Population and Housing.*

48. APIDS; "Request for Application (RFA)."

49. APIDS.

50. Ibid.

51. Wise, "Focus Group."

52. Lovely, "CO-99–12 Population Estimates."

53. Lipscomb interview, 2008.

54. Ibid.

55. Ibid.

56. Lipscomb interview, 2008.

57. Ibid.

58. For more on this population, see Edwards, Iritani, and Hallfors, "Prevalence and Correlates of Exchanging Sex."

59. Schable, Diaz, and Ward, "Epidemiology of HIV in the Rural South"; Cohn et al., "Geography of AIDS"; Davis, Cameron, and Stapleton. "Impact of HIV Patient Migration"; Rumley et al., "AIDS in Rural Eastern North Carolina."

60. Rumley et al., "AIDS in Rural Eastern North Carolina." In 1983, the indigenous rural cases were in Rowan, Lenoir, and Edgecombe counties. In 1984, indigenous cases surfaced in Wayne, Union, Craven, Sampson, Hertford, and Johnston counties. Finally, in 1985, indigenous rural cases appeared in Nash, Moore, Onslow, Wilson, Yadkin, Scotland, Richmond, Granville, Cleveland, Iredell, Watauga, Catawba, Davidson, McDowell, Robeson, Rutherford, and Pasquotank counties. See North Carolina Department of Health and Human Services, "North Carolina HIV Cases."

61. CDC, "Update: Trends in AIDS"; Lam and Liu, "Spread of AIDS." AIDS rates in communities with a population of between 50,000 and 500,000 and over 500,000 increased 3.3 percent and 3.1 percent, respectively.

62. Rumley et al., "AIDS in Rural Eastern North Carolina."

63. Ibid.

64. Womble, "Program Provides Fun and Education"; Wilson, "Dogwood Consortium." The nine counties were Cumberland, Harnett, Bladen, Robeson, Sampson, Hoke, Scotland, Columbus, and Duplin.

65. Rumley interview.

66. Ibid.

67. Rumley initially started an M.D./Ph.D. program at UNC but opted not to finish his Ph.D. program because of the duration of the program.

68. Rumley interview.

69. Ibid.

70. Ibid.

71. Ibid.

72. Ibid.

73. Ibid.

74. Ibid.

75. Ibid.

76. Ibid.

77. Ibid.

78. Rumley et al., "AIDS in Rural Eastern North Carolina."

79. Rumley, "Future of a Futureless Future."

80. Thomas, "From Slavery to Incarceration"; Adimora et al., "Concurrent Partnerships among Rural African Americans." Sixty percent of respondents reported never using condoms with their main partner; 9 percent recalled consistent condom use in the previous three months; 69 percent of men and 39 percent of women reported multiple sex partners in the previous three months. These numbers topped the rates of risky sex in urban communities, and 60 percent of rural respondents reported concurrent relationships (compared to 38 percent statewide). Moreover, Thomas believed the limited recall by respondents in Wilson County suggested substantially lower condom use. On sexually transmitted diseases in rural populations, see Thomas et al., "Syphilis in the South"; and Thomas et al., "Rural Gonorrhea."

81. Rumley interview.

82. Thomas and Gaffield, "Social Structure"; Kilmarx et al., "Ecologic Analysis"; Thomas, "From Slavery to Incarceration"; Thomas and Thomas, "Things Ain't What They Ought to Be."

83. Whetten-Goldstein and Nguyen, *You're the First One I've Told*, 33–36.

84. Ibid., 98.

85. Rumley interview.

86. Ibid.

87. Ibid.

88. Ibid.

89. Ibid.

90. Ibid.

91. van der Horst interview, 1998.

92. Rumley interview.

93. Ibid.

94. Rumley et al., "AIDS in Rural Eastern North Carolina."

95. Rumley interview

96. Ibid.

97. Rumley et al., "AIDS in Rural Eastern North Carolina."

98. Rumley interview; Jolly interview, November 8, 2007.

99. Rumley interview.

100. Ibid.

101. Jolly interview, November 8, 2007.

102. Rumley interview.

103. Ibid.

104. Ibid.

105. Ibid.

106. Ibid.

107. Ibid.

108. Ibid.

109. Ibid.

110. Ibid.

111. Ibid.

112. Rumley, "Future of a Futureless Future."

Chapter 6

1. Clabby, "AIDS Council."

2. North Carolina Department of Health and Human Services, Division of Public Health, HIV/STD Prevention and Care Branch, *N.C. Epidemiologic Profile* (2005), 18–19.

3. North Carolina AIDS Advisory Council, *NC/AIDS Index*. See also Associated Press, "Council"; Garloch, "N.C., 9,000 Test Positive for HIV"; and Steadman, "N.C. Leads Neighbors."

4. Zimmer, "AIDS Funding Evades State Budget Cuts." The federal poverty level for an individual in 1987 was $5,778. See Poverty and Health Statistics Branch/HHES Division, *Current Population Survey.*

5. Rumley interview.

6. Kirkpatrick, "Cost of AIDS Drugs."

7. General Assembly of North Carolina, 1993 Session, Ratified Bill, Chapter 321, Senate Bill 27. See also General Assembly of North Carolina, 1993 Session, Senate Bill 695/House Bill 738. See Kirkpatrick, "Drugs Elusive for 22 here."

8. Kirkpatrick, "Drugs Elusive for 22 Here"; Roslyn Savitt, *1995 North Carolina General Assembly Session, Legislative Report* (Raleigh: North Carolina HIV-AIDS Alliance, August 1995), Box 10, LGHP Records.

9. Even before protease inhibitors became available, several alternative Nucleoside-analogue Reverse Transcriptase Inhibitors (NRTIs) were available to clinicians. Between 1987 and 1998, six different NRTIs and one combination therapy came to the market: zidovudine, didanosine, zalcitabine, stavudine, lamivudine, abacavir, and Combivir (zidovudine and lamivudine). See "New AIDS Treatment Approved"; Associated Press, "FDA Approves DDC"; Recer, "Study: Drugs Other than AZT"; and Kirkpatrick, "Drugs Elusive for 22 here."

10. Clabby, "AIDS Council"; "AIDS Alarms."

11. North Carolina AIDS Advisory Council, *NC/AIDS Index.*

12. Clabby, "AIDS Council"; Associated Press, "Council"; Steadman, "N.C. Leads Neighbors."

13. Zimmer, "AIDS Moving Up on List".

14. Lamme, "Protease Inhibitor 'Brew' Offers Hope."

15. Rumley interview.

16. Ready, "New Drugs Brighten Prognosis for AIDS"; Schultz, "AIDS House Brimming with Health."

17. Schultz, "AIDS House Brimming with Health."

18. Lamme, "Protease Inhibitor 'Brew' Offers Hope."

19. Ready, "New Drugs Brighten Prognosis for AIDS."

20. Connor and Ho, "Human Immunodeficiency Virus Type 1 Variants"; Ho et al., "Rapid Turnover of Plasma Virions"; Ho, "Time to Hit HIV."

21. Ho, "Time to Hit HIV"; Ready, "New Drugs Brighten Prognosis for AIDS."

22. Lamme, "Care Lags Behind AIDS' Pace."

23. Ibid.

24. See Susan Sachs, "David Doss, Annie Dornberg Letter, May 16, 1995," Box 2, Correspondence, 1990–95, LGHP Records; Susan Sachs, "Jeff Prince Letter, September 22, 1995," Box 10, Community Connection, Piedmont Consortium, LGHP Records; and Susan Sachs, "Carolyn Harley Letter, October 16, 1995," Box 6, PHHC, 1991–95, LGHP Records.

25. Lamme, "Care Lags Behind AIDS' Pace."

26. Ibid.

27. Quigley, "AIDS Finds Victims with Rural Address." The four counties in the Cape Fear region with HIV/AIDS clinics were Sampson, Scotland, Columbus, and Cumberland.

28. Thomas, "From Slavery to Incarceration."

29. Zimmer, "Science Brings Hope."

30. Ibid.

31. Steadman, "N.C. Leads Neighbors."

32. Schmalz, "Whatever Happened to AIDS?"

33. Lamme, "Care Lags Behind AIDS' Pace."

34. Fulghum, "AIDS"; "HIV Infection to Be Monitored."

35. Jolly interview, November 8, 2007; Seymore, "AIDS Testing Change Barred"; Ross, "Anonymous Testing of AIDS Will Continue."

36. Seymore, "AIDS Testing Change Barred"; Alison Jones, "State Loses AIDS Test Suit"; "AIDS Secrecy."

37. Neergaard, "Officials Debate Whether HIV Patients Should Be Named."

38. Rhee, "Hunt's Agenda"; "Health Director Backs 'Confidential' HIV Tests." In the counties stopping anonymous testing, HIV tests of gay men dropped 11 percent.

39. "Health Director Backs 'Confidential' HIV Tests"; Associated Press, "AIDS Group to Fight for Anonymous Test Method"; Clark and Hagigh, "State Commission Ends Anonymous AIDS Tests"; Ready, "Judge Halts Plan to End Anonymous AIDS Tests"; Garloch, "Judge: Anonymous AIDS Testing Stays"; Nagy, "Anonymous Tests Win Reprieve."

40. Associated Press, "Commission Votes to End Anonymous HIV Testing."

41. Zimmer, "Activists Angry over HIV Testing Decision"; Zimmer, "Activists, N.C. Officials Meet in Court"; "Court Rules against Anonymous AIDS Tests"; Zimmer, "Court Ends Anonymous Test for HIV"; Zimmer, "Anonymous HIV Testing Gets Reprieve"; Zimmer, "N.C. Supreme Court to Rule on HIV Testing"; Zimmer, "Anonymous HIV Testing Heading to State Supreme Court"; Zimmer, "Court Ruling Spells End to Anonymous HIV Testing."

42. Jolly interview, November 8, 2007.

43. Moose, "Women and AIDS."

44. Lekus, "Health Care."

45. At the annual fund-raiser, for example, LGHP was only able to raise $2,000. Its counterparts in the joint fund-raising event raised $20,000 and $48,000, respectively. Even the local interfaith AIDS ministry raised more money than LGHP ($3,000). See "Minutes from NCLGHP Board Meeting, May 9, 1995," Box 1, Board Packets, 1995, LGHP Records. On the limited program offerings, see Minora Sharpe, "Letter to the Board of Directors, September 19, 1995," Box 1, Board Packets, 1995, LGHP Records; Jerry Harris, "Reducing Our Risks Update Letter to Bernadette Carr, June 1, 1995," Box 7, Reducing Our Risk, SRE, 1989–95, LGHP Records; Bernadette Carr, "Jerry Harris Letter, June 5, 1995," Box 7, Reducing Our Risk, SRE, 1989–95, LGHP Records; and Lekus, "Health Care."

46. Susan Sachs, "David Doss, Annie Dornberg Letter, May 16, 1995," Box 2, Correspondence, 1990–95, LGHP Records.

47. Susan Sachs, "Jeff Prince Letter, September 22, 1995," Box 10, Community Connection, Piedmont Consortium, LGHP Records.

48. Susan Sachs, "Carolyn Harley Letter, October 16, 1995," Box 6, PHHC, 1991–95, LGHP Records.

49. Harrison, "LGHP Ends Search for Director."

50. LGHP, "The North Carolina Lesbian and Gay Health Project: Emergency Board Meeting, October 10, 1995," Box 1, Board Packets, 1995, LGHP Records.

51. North Carolina AIDS Advisory Council, NC/AIDS Index. See also Lekus, "Health Care"; and Jolly interview, November 8, 2007.

52. Jolly interview, November 8, 2007; Levine interview.

53. General Assembly of North Carolina, Session 1995 [April 11, 1995], H834-CSRH-0045, "Teach Abstinence Until Marriage," Box 12, LGHP Records; Jim Watts and Robin Johnson, "Frances Cummings Memorandum, April 25, 1995," Box 12, LGHP Records; Roslyn Savitt, "North Carolina HIV-AIDS Alliance, 1995 North Carolina General Assembly Session, Legislative Report [August 1995]," 6–7, Box 10, LGHP Records; "Schools Must Teach Abstinence."

54. McLaughlin, "Guilford Schools Still Reviewing Sex Ed Materials"; Reale, "HIV Class Plays to Students' Interests."

55. Clabby, "Black Churches Reach out to AIDS Patients."

56. Garfield "New Year's Eve Given a Sacred Flavor"; Garfield, "Charlotte AIDS Fight Targets Black Ministers," 1C.

57. Johnston, "Black Churches to Join in AIDS Awareness Week."

58. Stocking, "Black Pastors Being Recruited"; Atwater, "Week of Prayer Promotes AIDS Ministry."

59. Bingham, "AIDS Battled from Pulpit"; Sharon E. White, "Living in the Shadow of AIDS"; Sharon E. White, "Week of Prayer for AIDS Healing."

60. Atwater, "Week of Prayer Promotes AIDS Ministry."

61. Jameson, "Delivering a Message about AIDS."

62. Fischer-Krentz, "Grants Awarded to Support Black Community"; "SCDAP to Implement Program for HIV-AIDS"; "Sickle Cell Grant."

63. CDC, AIDS Public Information Data Set (hereafter APIDS).

64. Ibid., compared to U.S. Census data.

65. Ibid., compared to U.S. Census data.

66. Ibid., compared to U.S. Census data.

67. These access differences were small but nonetheless noted in Gebo et al., "Racial and Gender Disparities."

68. Weslowski, Andrulis, and Martin, *AIDS in Rural America.*

69. Bonnie Wilson, "AIDS In County Rise By 57%"

70. Whyte and Carr, "Comparison of AIDS in Women."

71. Reif, Whetten, and Theilman, "Association of Race and Gender."

72. Cohn et al., "Care of HIV-Infected Adults"; Turner and Ball, "Variations in Inpatient Mortality"; Kitahata et al., "Physicians' Experience with the Acquired Immunodeficiency Syndrome"; Kitahata, Van Rompaey, and Shields, "Physician Experience in the Care of HIV-Infected Persons."

73. Crystal et al., "Initiation and Continuation of Newer Antiretroviral Treatments."

74. Quigley, "AIDS Finds Victims with Rural Address"; Thomas, "From Slavery to Incarceration."

75. Reif, Whetten, and Theilman, "Association of Race and Gender." See also Gebo et al., "Racial and Gender Disparities."

76. Heckman et al., "Barriers to Care"; McKinney, "Variations in Rural AIDS Epidemiology."

77. Rumley et al., "AIDS in Rural Eastern North Carolina"; Mainous and Matheny, "Rural Human Immunodeficiency Virus Health Service Provision"; Rounds, "AIDS in Rural Areas"; Blazer et al., "Health Services Access"; Aral, O'Leary, and Baker, "Sexually Transmitted Infections and HIV."

78. Rumley et al., "AIDS in Rural Eastern North Carolina"; Quigley, "AIDS Finds Victims with Rural Address."

79. Verghese, *My Own Country.* For more on AIDS stigma in North Carolina and across the South, see Aral, O'Leary, and Baker, "Sexually Transmitted Infections and HIV"; and "HIV/AIDS in Rural America."

80. Whetten-Goldstein and Nguyen, *"You're the First One I've Told,"* 102.

81. Ibid., 99.

82. Ibid., 102–3.

83. Golin et al., "Secret Pills."

84. Ibid.

85. Whetten-Goldstein and Nguyen, *"You're the First One I've Told,"* 100–101.

86. Maschal, "More Women Battle AIDS."

87. Whetten-Goldstein and Nguyen, *"You're the First One I've Told,"* 103.

88. CDC, *Drug-Associated HIV Transmission Continues in the United States,* cited in Southern State AIDS Directors Work Group, *Southern States Manifesto.*

89. Kaiser Commission on Medicaid and the Uninsured, *Medicaid Resource Book,* cited in Southern State AIDS Directors Work Group, *Southern States Manifesto.*

90. Southern State AIDS Directors Work Group, *Southern States Manifesto.*

91. Ibid.

92. The other three staffers were Phyllis Cochran, Brenda Crowder-Gaines, and Steve Sherman. See Southern State AIDS Directors Work Group, *Southern States Manifesto,* 3.

93. Comments of Steven Cline in Kaiser Family Foundation, National Alliance of State and Territorial AIDS Directors, and the Southern State AIDS Directors Work Group, "Southern States Summit on HIV/AIDS and STDs," 3.

94. Kaiser Family Foundation, National Alliance of State and Territorial AIDS Directors, and the Southern State AIDS Directors Work Group, "Southern States Summit on HIV/AIDS and STDs," 9.

95. Foust, "Call to Action."

96. Southern State AIDS Directors Work Group, *Southern States Manifesto.*

97. Ibid., 22–31.

98. Ibid., 11, 33.

99. Lichtenstein, Hook, and Sharma, "Public Tolerance, Private Pain."

100. CDC, *HIV/AIDS Surveillance Report, 2006.*

101. Whetten-Goldstein, Nguyen, and Heald, "Characteristics of Individuals Infected with the Human Immunodeficiency Virus"; McKinney, *Rural HIV/AIDS;* Lichtenstein, Hook, and Sharma, "Public Tolerance, Private Pain"; Napravnik et al., "Factors Associated with Fewer Visits"; Kaiser Family Foundation, "Sexually Transmitted Diseases In America."

102. Aral, O'Leary, and Baker, "Sexually Transmitted Infections and HIV"; CDC, *Sexually Transmitted Disease Surveillance, 2006;* Napravnik et al., "Factors Associated with Fewer Visits"; Shapiro et al., "Variations in the Care of HIV-Infected Adults"; Lichtenstein, "Stigma as a Barrier to Treatment"; Commonwealth Fund Commission, *Aiming Higher;* Lichtenstein, Hook, and Sharma, "Public Tolerance, Private Pain"; Anthony et al., *Access and Availability of HIV Testing and Treatment Services.*

103. Lichtenstein, Hook, and Sharma, "Public Tolerance, Private Pain"; Lichtenstein "Stigma as a Barrier to Treatment."

104. CDC, *HIV/AIDS Surveillance Report, 2006.*

105. Southern AIDS Coalition, *Southern States Manifesto.*

106. "HIV/AIDS Policy Fact Sheet."

107. Southern AIDS Coalition, *Southern States Manifesto,* 3.

108. Southern State AIDS Directors Work Group, *Southern States Manifesto,* 13.

109. Ricketts, *Rural Health in the United States*, cited in Southern State AIDS Directors Work Group, *Southern States Manifesto*, 14.

110. CDC, *HIV/AIDS Surveillance Report, 2005*.

111. Southern AIDS Coalition, *Southern States Manifesto*, 14.

112. Ibid., 16.

113. CDC, "Revised Recommendations for HIV Testing."

114. Clinicians and researchers now know symptoms can take a decade to develop after infection; in the early years of the epidemic, however, it was unclear whether an asymptomatic person testing positive for HIV antibodies would develop AIDS at all. As more people became sick, it became increasingly clear that people testing positive for HIV antibodies retained the virus, remained infectious, and would likely develop AIDS if left untreated (although there are some "non-progressors," that is, those who have the virus but never seem to develop AIDS or do so only after an extended period of time). During the period when researchers were collecting evidence for this, however, activists and clinicians differed significantly about what prognosis one could make from a positive test, and what the best response should be.

115. CDC, "Revised Recommendations for HIV Testing."

116. Southern AIDS Coalition, *Southern States Manifesto*.

117. Ibid., 3.

118. Southern AIDS Coalition, *2009–2010 HIV/AIDS Health Care Policy Brief and Recommendations*.

119. Southern AIDS Coalition, *Southern States Manifesto*, 14.

120. North Carolina Department of Health and Human Services, Division of Public Health, HIV/STD Prevention and Care Branch, "Get Real. Get Tested."

121. Southern AIDS Coalition, *Southern States Manifesto*, 14.

122. Fitzsimon, "Evelyn Foust on Combating AIDS in NC."

123. Fitzsimon, "Life-Threatening Budget Cuts."

124. North Carolina Department of Health and Human Services, Division of Public Health, Department of Communicable Disease, *N.C. Epidemiologic Profile* (2009), 94.

125. Ibid.

126. North Carolina Department of Health and Human Services, Division of Public Health, HIV/STD Prevention and Care Branch, HIV/STD Prevention and Care, *N.C. Epidemiologic Profile* (2007).

127. Ibid. The CDC's *HIV/AIDS Surveillance Report, 2008* actually showed that, from 2004 to 2007, HIV diagnoses increased 15 percent in the thirty-four states that had long-term, name-based HIV reporting. The CDC attributed these increases to four main factors: a) changes in state reporting regulations, b) more people getting tested, c) instability in the data, and d) actual increases in new HIV infections. Some or all of these factors may have been at work in the overall rising numbers. See CDC, "Questions and Answers."

128. North Carolina Department of Health and Human Services, Division of Public Health, HIV/STD Prevention and Care Branch, HIV/STD Prevention and Care, *N.C. Epidemiologic Profile* (2007).

129. Ibid.

130. According to the Division of Public Health's HIV/STD Prevention and Care Branch, "HIV was not consistently reported in all states; thus the region/state HIV (not AIDS) comparisons are only for those states that reported HIV" (ibid., 24).

131. Ibid.

132. North Carolina Department of Health and Human Services, Division of Public Health, Department of Communicable Disease, *N.C. Epidemiologic Profile* (2009), 92.

133. CDC, "Adoption of Protective Behaviors," and Palella et al., "Survival Benefits of Initiating Antiretroviral Therapy," cited in North Carolina Department of Health and Human Services, Division of Public Health, Department of Communicable Disease, *N.C. Epidemiologic Profile* (2009), 92.

134. North Carolina Department of Health and Human Services, Division of Public Health, HIV/STD Prevention and Care Branch, HIV/STD Prevention and Care, *N.C. Epidemiologic Profile* (2007).

135. North Carolina Department of Health and Human Services, Division of Public Health, Department of Communicable Disease, *N.C. Epidemiologic Profile* (2009), 91.

136. Ibid.

137. Ibid., 91–92.

138. Ibid.

139. Ibid.

140. Ibid., 93.

Conclusion

1. Copley, *Watson and the Shark.*

2. Rumley interview.

3. 1984 and 2000 rankings from CDC, AIDS Public Information Data Set; 2007 data from CDC, "Basic Statistics."

4. van der Horst interview, 1998.

5. Marston and King, "Factors that Shape Young People's Sexual Behaviour."

6. Southern State AIDS/STD Directors Work Group, "Southern States Manifesto," 16.

7. Ford et al., "Black Sexuality."

8. Ibid.

9. Ibid. North Carolina's experience seems to contradict, or at least complicate, Ford et al.'s argument at this point.

10. For a greater discussion of multiple marginalization, see Cathy J. Cohen, *Boundaries of Blackness.*

11. Ford et al., "Black Sexuality."

12. Bayer, *Private Acts, Social Consequences,* 260–61.

13. Lichtenstein, Hook, and Sharma, "Public Tolerance, Private Pain."

14. Bayer, *Private Acts, Social Consequences,* 260–61.

15. For more on some of these criticisms, see Gostin, "Public Health Law."

16. For more on this, see Neumann and Sogolow, "Replicating Effective Programs"; Resnicow et al., "Cultural Sensitivity in Public Health"; and Ortiz-Torres, Serrano-García, and Torres-Burgos, "Subverting Culture."

17. Thomas and Torrone, "Incarceration as Forced Migration."

18. Rumley, "Future of a Futureless Future."

19. Nietzsche, *Beyond Good and Evil*.

BIBLIOGRAPHY

Primary Sources

MANUSCRIPT COLLECTIONS
Chapel Hill, N.C.
  Southern Oral History Program Collection #4007, Center for the Study
      of the American South, University of North Carolina, Chapel Hill
    Oral History Interview by Cecil W. Wooten, July 16, 2001, Interview
      K-0849
Durham, N.C.
  Rare Book, Manuscript, and Special Collections Library, Duke University
      North Carolina Council of Churches Records
    North Carolina Lesbian and Gay Health Project Records, 1983–1996
Ithaca, N.Y.
  Division of Rare and Manuscript Collections, Cornell University Library
      National Lesbian and Gay Health Association Records

INTERVIEWS
Adinolfi, Anthony. Interview by author, Durham, N.C., November 28, 2007.
Alston, Louise. Interview by author, Durham, N.C., March 28, 2008.
Duvall, Jill. Interview by Ian Lekus, Durham, N.C., March 2, 1994.
Fitts, Howard. Interview by author, Durham, N.C., March 17, 2008.
Hamilton, John. Interview by author, Durham, N.C., November 2005.
Hart-Brothers, Elaine. Interview by author, Durham, N.C., April 2008.
Herndon, Godfrey. Interview by author, Durham, N.C., February 8, 2006.
———. Interview by Ian Lekus, Durham, N.C., June 2, 1994.
Jolly, David. Interview by author, Durham, N.C., November 8, 2007.
———. Interview by author, Durham, N.C., December 21, 2007.
Jones, David. Interview by Ian Lekus, Durham, N.C., February 23, 1994.
Lee, Lester. Interview by Ian Lekus, Durham, N.C., June 1, 1994.
Levine, Ronald. Interview by author, Durham, N.C., November 19, 2007.
Lipscomb, Garry. Interview by author, Durham, N.C., March 27, 2008.
———. Interview by Ian Lekus, Durham, N.C., May 23, 1994.
Noto, Dante. Interview by Ian Lekus, Durham, N.C., February 11, 1994.
———. Interview by author, San Francisco, Calif., November 1, 2007.
Rumley, Richard L. Interview by author, Greenville, N.C., May 2010.
Rutherford, Carleton. Interview by author, Durham, N.C., May 30, 2008.

Smiley, Lynn. Interview by author, Chapel Hill, N.C., November 29, 2007.
van der Horst, Charles. Interview by Ronald Bayer, New York City, June 3, 1998.
————. Interview by author, Chapel Hill, N.C., December 3, 2007.

Secondary Sources

Ackerman, Sara, Christopher Allen, Elisa Gladstone, Vanya Jones, Jeffrey Novey, Sara Reddy, and Xan Young. "The Triangle Lesbian, Gay, Bisexual, and Transgender Community, Wake, Durham, and Orange Counties, North Carolina: A Community Diagnosis Including Secondary Data Analysis and Qualitative Data Collection." Master's thesis. University of North Carolina School of Public Health, 1999.

Adelman, Robert M., Chris Morett, and Stewart E. Tolnay. "Homeward Bound: The Return Migration of Southern-Born Black Women, 1940 to 1990." *Sociological Spectrum* 20 (2000): 433–63.

Adimora, A. A., V. Schoenbach, D. Bonas, F. Martinson, K. Donaldson, and T. Stancil. "Concurrent Sexual Partnerships among Women in the United States." *Epidemiology* 13 (2002): 320–27.

Adimora, Adaora A., and Victor J. Schoenbach. "Social Context, Sexual Networks, and Racial Disparities in Rates of Sexually Transmitted Infections." *Journal of Infectious Diseases* 191 (2005): S115–S122.

Adimora, Adaora A., Victor J. Schoenbach, Francis Martinson, Kathryn H. Donaldson, Tonya R. Stancil, and Robert E. Fullilove. "Concurrent Sexual Partnerships among African Americans in the Rural South." *Annals of Epidemiology* 14 (3) (March 2004): 155–60.

————. "Concurrent Partnerships among Rural African Americans with Recently Reported Heterosexually Transmitted HIV Infection." *Journal of Acquired Immune Deficiency Syndromes* 34 (4) (2003): 423–29.

Advisory Committee for HIV and STD Prevention. "HIV Prevention through Early Detection and Treatment of Other Sexually Transmitted Diseases—United States Recommendations of the Advisory Committee for HIV and STD Prevention." *MMWR* 47 (RR12) (July 31, 1998): 1–24.

"AIDS: Its Impact on Women, Children, and Families, June 12, 1987." Public Hearing. New York State Division on Women, 1987.

"AIDS Alarms." *Raleigh News & Observer*, December 4, 1996.

"AIDS and Migrant Workers." *Boston Globe*, September 9, 1988, 18.

"AIDS Cases in N.C. Multiplying at 3 Times the National Rate." *Fayetteville Observer*, May 18, 1990.

"AIDS Cases Swamping N.C. Prisons." *Charlotte Observer*, May 16, 1990, 2B.

"AIDS Education Question." *Charlotte Observer*, January 12, 1987, 2D.

"AIDS Fight Deserves Support." *North Carolina Independent*, June 24, 1983.

"AIDS News Update: Falwell's Claim of 'God's Judgment' Hit by N.Y.'s Bishop Moore." *Advocate*, July 1983.

"AIDS Secrecy." *Fayetteville Observer*, June 7, 1993.

"AIDS Threat Growing among Women." *Greensboro News & Record*, November 30, 1990, A7.

"AIDS Warning Splits Doctors." *Charlotte Observer*, July 4, 1988, 2B.

Allegood, Jerrey. "AIDS: 24 Hours on the Front Line." *Raleigh News & Observer*, September 16, 1990, A1, 12–13.

Allen, Patti, and John Koepke. "Look Back: Transfusion-Acquired HIV Infection at Duke University Medical Center." *North Carolina Medical Journal* 49 (12) (December 1988): 657–61.

Altman, Dennis. *AIDS in the Mind of America: The Social, Political, and Psychological Impact of a New Epidemic.* Garden City, N.Y.: Anchor Books, 1987.

Alvarado, Donna. "AIDS Victims Physically Devastated, Socially Isolated." *Raleigh News and Observer*, February 2, 1986, 27A.

———. "Doctors Urged: Take All AIDS You Can." *Raleigh Times*, November 12, 1987, 3D.

———. "Durham Victim Draws Strength from Family," *Raleigh News & Observer*, August 4, 1985, 1D.

———. "Easing Public's Fear of AIDS While Guarding Patient Rights." *Raleigh News and Observer*, June 15, 1986, 1D, 5D.

"AMA Says Tracing Could Fight AIDS." *Charlotte Observer*, July 1, 1988, 19A.

Anderson, R. M. "Transmission Dynamics of Sexually Transmitted Infections." In *Sexually Transmitted Diseases*, 3rd ed., edited by K. K. Holmes, P. A. Mardh, P. F. Sparling et al., 25–37. New York: McGraw-Hill, 1999.

"Anonymous AIDS Testing on Agenda." *Charlotte Observer*, November 8, 1989, 3C.

"Anonymous AIDS Tests Assured." *Charlotte Observer*, November 10, 1989, 1B.

Anthony, M. N., M. Sutton, C. Vila, S. D. Holmbert, V. Gol, E. McLellan-Lemal, L. Fitzpatrick, M. S. Matthew, L. A. Crandall, and P. J. Weidle. *Access and Availability of HIV Testing and Treatment Services in U.S. Southern Rural Counties.* Atlanta, Ga.: National HIV Prevention Conference, December 2007.

Aral, S. O. "The Social Context of Syphilis Persistence in the Southeastern United States." *Sexually Transmitted Diseases* 23 (1) (1996): 9–15.

Aral, S. O., A. A. Adimora, and K. A. Fenton. "Understanding and Responding to Disparities in HIV and Other Sexually Transmitted Infections in African Americans." *Lancet* 372 (9635) (2008): 337–40.

Aral, Sevgi O., Ann O'Leary, and Charlene Baker. "Sexually Transmitted Infections and HIV in the Southern United States: An Overview." *Sexually Transmitted Diseases* 33 (7 Supplement) (July 2006): S1–S5.

Arrington, Fran. "Displaced Children Have No Place to Go: Social Services Trying to Help Orphans of Addiction." *Raleigh News & Observer*, November 18, 1991, B1.

———. "IV-Drug Use Injects Durham with New Wave of Problems." *Raleigh News & Observer*, December 21, 1991, B3.

Associated Press. "AIDS Bill." *Charlotte Observer*, February 8, 1989, 5B.

———. "AIDS Case May Alter Transplant Policies." *Charlotte Observer*, September 9, 1986, 2C.

————. "AIDS Education Bill Filed in House." *Charlotte Observer*, April 16, 1987, 3C.

————. "AIDS Education Plan Downplays Condoms." *Charlotte Observer*, December 3, 1987, 4C.

————. "AIDS Group to Fight for Anonymous Test Method." *Charlotte Observer*, June 16, 1994, 3C.

————. "AIDS-Patient Confidentiality Puts Doctors in Bind." *Charlotte Observer*, September 14, 1987, 3B.

————. "Commission Votes to End Anonymous HIV Testing." *Durham Herald-Sun*, February 10, 1995, C5.

————. "Council: HIV-Positive Tar Heels May Be Double Reported Figure." *Durham Herald-Sun*, December 3, 1996, C12.

————. "Division Seeks Reporting Rule on AIDS Cases." *Raleigh Times*, July 1983.

————. "FDA Approves DDC as a Single-Drug Treatment for AIDS Virus Infection." *Charlotte Observer*, August 9, 1994, 4A.

————. "Gonorrhea, Syphilis on Rise in N.C. Increase Is Blamed on People Exchanging Sex for Drugs." *Charlotte Observer*, November 7, 1991, 2C.

————. "Group Seeks Donations for AIDS House." *Charlotte Observer*, April 16, 1988.

————. "Martin: AIDS Focus Should Be on Abstinence." *Charlotte Observer*, September 25, 1987, 1D.

————. "Migrants' Poor Health Blamed on Isolation." *Charlotte Observer*, September 2, 1987, 2B.

————. "N.C. House Accepts Senate's Version of Bill on AIDS." *Charlotte Observer*, August 12, 1987, 8E.

————. "N.C. House Rejects Mandatory AIDS Tests." *Charlotte Observer*, May 27, 1987, 2B.

————. "N.C. Legislature Must Act This Year to Contain AIDS Spread, Groups Say." *Charlotte Observer*, April 17, 1989, 2B.

————. "N.C. Seeks Grant for AIDS Programs." *Charlotte Observer*, August 23, 1987.

————. "New Definition Triples Number of N.C. AIDS Cases." *Charlotte Observer*, February 20, 1988, 1C.

————. "Panel Backs Elections between Presidential Races." *Charlotte Observer*, August 6, 1987, 4B.

————. "Prison Bills Might Avert Federal Action." *Charlotte Observer*, February 18, 1987, 2B.

————. "Senate Oks AIDS Legislation: Lawmakers Credit Changes House Made." *Charlotte Observer*, July 29, 1989, 12B.

————. "Senate OKs Revised AIDS Education Bill." *Charlotte Observer*, July 8, 1987, 3B.

————. "Six Received Blood Product Recalled over AIDS Threat." *Raleigh Times*, September 1, 1983, A24.

————. "State Survey Focuses on AIDS Problem in Prison." *Charlotte Observer*, November 3, 1989, 2D.

————. "States that Require AIDS Education in School Triple in Six Months." *New York Times*, December 4, 1987, B5.

———. "Study Indicates N.C. Migrant Workers Have High Rate of AIDS Infection." *Charlotte Observer*, September 2, 1988, 1E.

———. "Task Force Offers Final Proposal for AIDS Rules." *Charlotte Observer*, December 2, 1987, 1B.

———. "Workshop Focus: AIDS and Blacks Official Calls Economics a Major Factor in Crisis." *Charlotte Observer*, January 29, 1990, 12B.

Atwater, Jada Harris. "Week of Prayer Promotes AIDS Ministry in Black Churches." *Chapel Hill Herald*, March 3, 1996, 1.

"Avoid Demagoguery on AIDS." *Charlotte Observer*, January 21, 1988.

"Bad News Is Getting Worse U.S. Must Attack Causes of High Infant Mortality Rate." *Charlotte Observer*, March 4, 1990.

Baker, James N., and Regina Elam. "Joining the AIDS Fight." *Newsweek*, April 17, 1989, 26–27.

Ballard, Connie. "AIDS." *Raleigh Times*, May 26, 1983.

———. "AIDS: New Duke Clinic One of Signs of Growing Attention Being Paid to Mystery Disease." *Raleigh Times*, May 26, 1983, A1, B1.

Barré-Sinoussi, F., J. C. Chermann, F. Rey, M. T. Nugeyre, S. Chamaret, J. Gruest, C. Dauguet, C. Axler-Blin, F. Vézinet-Brun, C. Rouzioux, W. Rozenbaum, and L. Montagnier. "Isolation of a T-lymphotropic Retrovirus from a Patient at Risk for Acquired Immune Deficiency Syndrome (AIDS)." *Science* 220 (4599) (May 20, 1983): 868–71.

Bartlett, John. "HIV Testing in North Carolina." *North Carolina Medical Journal* 51 (4) (April 1990): 150–51.

Bayer, Ronald. "AIDS and the Making of an Ethics of Public Health." In *Dawning Answers: How the HIV/AIDS Epidemic Has Helped to Strengthen Public Health*, edited by Ronald O. Valdiserri, 135–54. New York: Oxford University Press, 2003.

———. "Clinical Progress and the Future of HIV Exceptionalism." *Archives of Internal Medicine* 139 (10) (1999): 1042–48.

———. "Entering the Second Decade: The Politics of Prevention, the Politics of Neglect." In *AIDS: The Making of a Chronic Disease*, edited by Elizabeth Fee and Daniel M. Fox, 207–26. Berkeley: University of California Press, 1992.

———. *Private Acts, Social Consequences: AIDS and the Politics of Public Health*. New Brunswick, N.J.: Rutgers University Press, 1989, 1991.

Bayer, Ronald, and Claire Edington. "HIV Testing, Human Rights, and Global AIDS Policy: Exceptionalism and Its Discontents." *Journal of Health Politics, Policy and Law* 34 (3) (June 2009): 304–7.

Bayer, Ronald, and David L. Kirp. "The United States: At the Center of the Storm." In *AIDS in the Industrialized Democracies*, edited by David L. Kirp and Ronald Bayer, 7–48. New Brunswick, N.J.: Rutgers University Press, 1992.

Bingham, Larry. "AIDS Battled from Pulpit." *Fayetteville Observer*, October 28, 1996.

Blazer, D. G., L. R. Landerman, G. Fillenbaum, and R. Horner. "Health Services Access and Use among Older Adults in North Carolina: Urban vs Rural Residents." *American Journal of Public Health* 85 (10) (October 1995): 1384–90.

"Bleak Future Seen for Poor with AIDS." *Charlotte Observer*, January 1, 1990, 4B.

Boyce, F. Alan. "Prisons Seek Aid for AIDS Rising Inmate Caseload Stretches Health Budget." *Charlotte Observer*, November 20, 1990, 1C.

Braithwaite, John. "The Irony of State Intervention: Labeling Theory." In *Criminological Theory: Context and Consequences*, edited by J. Robert Lilly, Francis T. Cullen, and Richard A. Ball, 123–48. Thousand Oaks, Calif.: Sage, 2007.

Bronski, Michael. "Carnival as Organizing." *Z Magazine*, April 2004.

Brown, Tony, Dean Smith, and Diane Suchetka. "How Safe Is Sex?" *Charlotte Observer*, November 21, 1991, 1E.

Buechler, Steven. *Social Movements in Advanced Capitalism*. New York: Oxford University Press, 1999.

Burch, Mary. "Dead Inmate Is AIDS Victim." *Raleigh Times*, May 28, 1983.

Buse, Kent, Nicholas Mays, and Gill Walt. *Making Health Policy*. New York: Open University Press, 2005.

Califano, Joseph A., Jr. "Three-Headed Dog from Hell: The Staggering Public Health Threat Posed by AIDS, Substance Abuse and Tuberculosis." *Washington Post*, December 21, 1992, A21.

Calonge, B. N., L. R. Petersen, R. S. Miller, and G. Marshall. "Human Immunodeficiency Virus Seroprevalence in Primary Care Practices in the United States." *Western Journal of Medicine* 158 (2) (1993): 148–52.

Campbell, Carole. *Women, Families, & HIV/AIDS: A Sociological Perspective on the Epidemic in America*. New York: Cambridge University Press, 1999.

Carlson, Bonnie. "AIDS Home." *Fayetteville Observer*, March 13, 1995.

"Carl Wittman." *The Knitting Circle*, London South Bank University, August 11, 1999 (cited November 4, 2005), http://myweb.lsbu.ac.uk/~stafflag/carlwittman.html.

"Carolinas Cases: A Glimpse of the Faces behind the Statistics." *Charlotte Observer*, June 5, 1983, 10.

Catanoso, Justin. "Confidential AIDS Testing Divides Health Community." *Greensboro News & Record*, February 3, 1991, A1.

Centers for Disease Control and Prevention. "Adoption of Protective Behaviors among Persons with Recent HIV Infection and Diagnosis—Alabama, New Jersey, and Tennessee, 1997–1998." *MMWR* 49 (2000): 512–15.

———. AIDS Public Information Data Set (APIDS) U.S. Surveillance Data for 1981–2002. CDC WONDER On-line Database, December 2005.

———. AIDS Public Information Data Set (APIDS) U.S. Surveillance Data for 1981–2002, CDC WONDER Downloadable Database, software version 2.7.1, December 2005.

———. "Basic Statistics: AIDS Cases by Top 10 States/Dependent Areas," http://www.cdc.gov/hiv/topics/surveillance/basic.htm. April 1, 2009.

———. "Current Trends: Partner Notification for Preventing Human Immunodeficiency Virus (HIV) Infection—Colorado, Idaho, South Carolina, Virginia." *MMWR* 37 (25) (1988): 393–96, 401–2.

———. "Current Trends: Prevention of Acquired Immune Deficiency Syndrome

(AIDS): Report of Inter-Agency Recommendations" *MMWR* 32 (March 4, 1983): 101–3.

———. "Current Trends Update: Acquired Immunodeficiency Syndrome (AIDS)—United States." *MMWR* 32 (30) (August 5, 1983): 389–91.

———. *Drug-Associated HIV Transmission Continues in the United States*. Atlanta, Ga.: Centers for Disease Control and Prevention, 2002.

———. "Epidemiologic Notes and Reports *Pneumocystis Carinii* Pneumonia among Persons with Hemophilia A." *MMWR* 31 (27) (July 16, 1982): 365–67.

———. "Estimated Numbers of Adults and Adolescents Living with AIDS by Region, 1993–2007—50 States and DC, Slide 7." In *AIDS Surveillance—General Epidemiology (through 2007)*. Atlanta, Ga.: U.S. Department of Health and Human Services, Centers for Disease Control and Prevention, 2007, http://www.cdc.gov/hiv/topics/surveillance/resources/slides/epidemiology/index.htm. June 8, 2010.

———. *HIV/AIDS Surveillance Report, 2005*. Vol. 17, rev. ed. Atlanta, Ga.: Centers for Disease Control and Prevention, June 2007, http://www.cdc.gov/hiv/surveillance/resources/reports/2005report/. June 15, 2010.

———. *HIV/AIDS Surveillance Report, 2006*. Vol. 18. Atlanta, Ga.: U.S. Department of Health and Human Services, Centers for Disease Control and Prevention, 2008, http://www.cdc.gov/hiv/surveillance/resources/reports/2006report/. June 15, 2010.

———. *HIV/AIDS Surveillance Report, 2007*. Vol. 19. Atlanta, Ga.: U.S. Department of Health and Human Services, Centers for Disease Control and Prevention, 2009, http://www.cdc.gov/hiv/surveillance/resources/reports/2007report/. June 15, 2010.

———. *HIV/AIDS Surveillance Report, 2008*. Vol. 20. Atlanta, Ga.: U.S. Department of Health and Human Services, Centers for Disease Control and Prevention, 2010, http://www.cdc.gov/hiv/surveillance/resources/reports/2008report/. June 15, 2010.

———. "HIV Transmission among Black College Student and Non-Student Men Who Have Sex with Men—North Carolina, 2003." *MMWR* 53 (32) (August 20, 2004): 731–34.

———. "HIV Transmission among Black Women—-North Carolina, 2004." *MMWR* 54 (4) (February 4, 2005): 89–94.

———. "1992 National Health Interview Survey." In *Healthy People 2000 Review*. Washington, D.C.: U.S. Department of Health and Human Services, 1994.

———. "Possible Transfusion-Associated Acquired Immunodeficiency Syndrome (AIDS)—California." *MMWR* 31 (1982): 652–54.

———. "Proportions of AIDS Cases among Adults and Adolescents, by Race/Ethnicity and Year of Diagnosis 1985–2007—United States and Dependent Areas, Slide 2." In *HIV/AIDS Surveillance by Race/Ethnicity (through 2007)*. Washington, D.C.: U.S. Health and Human Services, April 10, 2009, http://www.cdc.gov/hiv/topics/surveillance/resources/slides/race-ethnicity/index.htm. June 8, 2010.

———. "Questions and Answers: The 15% Increase in HIV Diagnoses from 2004–2007 in 34 States and General Surveillance Report Questions." Atlanta, Ga.: Centers for Disease Control and Prevention, February 26, 2009, http://www.cdc.gov/hiv/topics/surveillance/resources/qa/surv_rep.htm. May 21, 2010.

———. "Revised Recommendations for HIV Testing of Adults, Adolescents, and Pregnant Women in Health-Care Settings." *MMWR* 55 (RR14) (September 22, 2006): 1–17.

———. *Sexually Transmitted Disease Surveillance, 2006.* Atlanta, Ga.: U.S. Department of Health and Human Services, November 2007, http://www.cdc.gov/std/stats/toc2006.htm. June 8, 2010.

———. "Update: Trends in AIDS among Men Who Have Sex with Men—United States, 1989–1994." *MMWR* 44 (21) (1995): 401–40.

Chambers, Joseph. "Let's Talk." *Charlotte Observer*, September 13, 1985.

Chandler, E. T. "The High Cost of Failure: Prisoners with and without HIV Infection." *North Carolina Medical Journal* 52 (6) (June 1991): 255–58.

Chen, Daniel L., and Jo Thori Lind. "The Political Economy of Beliefs: Why Fiscal and Social Conservatives and Liberals Come Hand-in-Hand." Paper presented at the annual meeting of the American Political Science Association, Philadelphia, Pa., August 31, 2006, http://www.allacademic.com/meta/p152217_index.html. June 11, 2010.

"Children with AIDS Seen as No Threat in Classroom." *Charlotte Observer*, January 19 1986.

"Churches and AIDS: Responsibilities in Mission." *Christianity and Crisis*, December 9, 1985, 483.

Ciesielski, S. D., J. R. Seed, D. H. Esposito, and N. Hunter. "The Epidemiology of Tuberculosis among North Carolina Migrant Farm Workers." *Journal of the American Medical Association* 265 (13) (1991): 1715–19.

"Civilian Labor Force Estimates for North Carolina, 1980–1990." Raleigh: Employment Security Commission of North Carolina, 2003.

Clabby, Catherine. "AIDS Council Wants Greater Emphasis on Prevention." *Raleigh News & Observer*, December 3, 1996, A3.

———. "Black Churches Reach out to AIDS Patients." *Raleigh News & Observer*, May 28, 1996, A1.

———. "State Testing Program Cuts Incidence of HIV." *Raleigh News & Observer*, May 15, 1996, B1.

Clark, Paul Coe, III, and Jaleh Hagigh. "State Commission Ends Anonymous AIDS Tests." *Raleigh News & Observer*, August 6, 1994, A3.

Clear, T. R., D. R. Rose, E. Waring, and K. Scully. "Coercive Mobility and Crime: A Preliminary Examination of Concentrated Incarceration and Social Disorganization." *Justice Quarterly* 20 (2003): 33–64.

Clemmons, C. J. "AIDS Outreach Called Frustrating, Necessary." *Charlotte Observer*, November 26, 1994, 1C.

Cohen, Cathy J. *The Boundaries of Blackness: AIDS and the Breakdown of Black Politics.* Chicago: University of Chicago Press, 1999.

Cohen, D., R. Scribner, J. Clark, and D. Cory. "The Potential Role of Custody Facilities in Controlling Sexually Transmitted Diseases." *American Journal of Public Health* 82 (1992): 552–56.

Cohen, Jon. *Shots in the Dark: The Wayward Search for an AIDS Vaccine.* New York: W. W. Norton, 2001.

Cohen, Myron S. "HIV and Sexually Transmitted Diseases: Lethal Synergy." *International AIDS Society–USA, Topics in HIV Medicine* 12 (4) (October/November 2004): 104–7.

Cohn, S. E., M. L. Berk, S. H. Berry, N. Duan, M. R. Frankel, J. D. Klein, M. M. McKinney, A. Rastegar, S. Smith, M. F. Shapiro, and S. A. Bozzette. "The Care of HIV-Infected Adults in Rural Areas of the United States." *Journal of Acquired Immune Deficiency Syndromes* 28 (4) (2001): 385–92.

Cohn, S. E., J. D. Klein, J. E. Mohr, C. M. van der Horst, and D. J. Weber. "The Geography of Aids: Patterns of Urban and Rural Migration." *Southern Medical Journal* 87 (6) (June 1994): 599–606.

Colwell, Sylvia. "Tracey Marshall's Message Lives On." *Charlotte Observer*, July 24, 1994, 4.

The Commonwealth Fund. *Aiming Higher: Results from a State Scorecard on Health System Performance, 2009; The Commowealth Fund Commission on a High Performance Health System.* New York: The Commonwealth Fund, 2009.

Connor, Edward M., Rhoda S. Sperling, Richard Gelber, Pavel Kiselev, Gwendolyn Scott, Mary Jo O'Sullivan, Russell VanDyke, Mohammed Bey, William Shearer, Robert L. Jacobson, Eleanor Jimenez, Edward O'Neill, Brigitte Bazin, Jean-Francois Delfraissy, Mary Culnane, Robert Coombs, Mary Elkins, Jack Moye, Pamela Stratton, and James Balsley for the Pediatric AIDS Clinical Trials Group Protocol 076 Study Group. "Reduction of Maternal-Infant Transmission of Human Immunodeficiency Virus Type 1 with Zidovudine Treatment. Pediatric AIDS Clinical Trials Group Protocol 076 Study Group." *New England Journal of Medicine* 331 (18) (November 3, 1994): 1173–80.

Connor, R. I., and D. D. Ho. "Human Immunodeficiency Virus Type 1 Variants with Increased Replicative Capacity Develop during the Asymptomatic Stage before Disease Progression." *Journal of Virology* 68 (7) (July 1994): 4400–408.

Connor, Steve, and Sharon Kingman. *The Search for the Virus: The Scientific Discovery of AIDS and the Quest for a Cure.* 2nd. ed. New York: Viking Penguin, 1989.

Cook, Robert L., Rachel A. Royce, James C. Thomas, and Barbara H. Hanusa. "What's Driving an Epidemic? The Spread of Syphilis Along an Interstate Highway in Rural North Carolina." *American Journal of Public Health* 89 (3) (March 1999): 369–73.

"Court Rules against Anonymous AIDS Tests." *Raleigh News & Observer*, June 10, 1995, B3.

Crase, Darrell, and Hollie Walker Jr. "Black Students and Professionals in Health Education." ERIC Microfiche Collection (ED292755), 1987.

Crystal, Stephen, Usha Sambamoorthi, Patrick J. Moynihan, and Elizabeth McSpiritt. "Initiation and Continuation of Newer Antiretroviral Treatments among Medicaid Recipients with AIDS." *Journal of General Internal Medicine* 16 (12) (January 12, 2002): 850–59.

Cunningham, Henry. "10-County Region Reports 89 Cases of AIDS since 1984." *Fayetteville Observer*, June 19, 1989.

Dalton, H. L. "AIDS in Blackface." *Daedalus* (Summer 1989): 205–27.

Daniels, N., B. P. Kennedy, and I. Kawachi. "Justice Is Good for Our Health." In *Is Inequality Bad for Our Health?*, edited by N. Daniels, B. P. Kennedy, I. Kawachi, 3–33. Boston: Beacon, 2000.

Darrow, W. W. "Venereal Infections in Three Ethnic Groups in Sacramento." *American Journal of Public Health* 66 (1976): 446–50.

Davidson, O. G. *Broken Heartland: The Rise of America's Rural Ghetto.* Iowa City: University of Iowa Press, 1996.

Davis, K. A., B. Cameron, and J. T. Stapleton. "The Impact of HIV Patient Migration to Rural Areas." *AIDS Patient Care and STDs* 6 (5) (1992): 225–28.

Department of Geography and Earth Sciences, University of North Carolina at Charlotte. The North Carolina Atlas Revisited, www.ncatlasrevisited.org.

Division of STD Prevention. *Sexually Transmitted Disease Surveillance, 2002.* Atlanta, Ga.: Centers for Disease Control and Prevention, September 2003.

"Doctor: Anonymous AIDS Test No Longer Serves Good Purpose." *Charlotte Observer,* February 4, 1991, 4B.

Dombey-Moore, B., S. Resetar, and M. Childress. *A System Description of the Cocaine Trade.* Santa Monica, Calif.: RAND, 1994.

Dombrowski, Julia C., James C. Thomas, and Jay S. Kaufman. "A Study in Contrasts: Measures of Racial Disparity in Rates of Sexually Transmitted Disease." *Sexually Transmitted Diseases* 31 (3) (March 2004): 149–53.

Drug Enforcement Administration. *Drug Enforcement Administration: A Tradition of Excellence, 1973–2003.* Washington, D.C.: Drug Enforcement Administration, 2003, 59–61, http://www.usdoj.gov/dea/pubs/history/history_part1.pdf.

Duffus, W., L. Kettinger, T. Stephens, J. Gibson, K. Weis, M. Tyrell, D. Patterson, C. Finney, W. P. Bailey, B. Branson, L. Gardner, and H. Kilmarx. "Missed Opportunities for Earlier Diagnosis of HIV Infection — South Carolina, 1997–2005." *MMWR* 55 (47) (December 1, 2006): 1269–72.

Durack, D. T. "Opportunistic Infections and Kaposi's Sarcoma in Homosexual Men." *New England Journal of Medicine,* December 10, 1981, 305.

Durham Committee Institute. "AIDS Risk Reduction/Minority Education Projects Quarterly Report." January 23, 1989. Howard Fitts Personal Collection, Durham, N.C.

———. "Clearinghouse and Network Center for AIDS Education." 1988. Howard Fitts Personal Collection, Durham, N.C.

———. "Clearinghouse and Network Center for AIDS Education, Quarterly Report (January 23, 1989)." Howard Fitts Personal Collection, Durham, N.C.

———. "Proposal: Clearinghouse and Network Center for AIDS Education among Minority Populations in Ten Piedmont and Eastern North Carolina Counties, June 14, 1988." Howard Fitts Personal Collection, Durham, N.C.

"Editorial." *Shelby Star*, August 29, 1983.

"Educators Denounce Brochure." *FrontPage*, June 26, 1992, 1, 8.

Edwards, J. M., B. J. Iritani, and D. D. Hallfors. "Prevalence and Correlates of Exchanging Sex for Drugs or Money among Adolescents in the United States." *Sexually Transmitted Infections* 82 (2006): 354–58.

"Epidemiologic Notes and Reports: HIV Seroprevalence in Migrant and Seasonal Farmworkers—North Carolina, 1987." *MMWR* 37 (34) (September 2, 1988): 517–19.

Epstein, Steven. *Impure Science: AIDS, Activism, and the Politics of Knowledge.* Berkeley, Calif.: University of California Press, 1996.

———. *Inclusion: The Politics of Difference in Medical Research.* Chicago: University of Chicago Press, 2007.

Evatt, B. "Infectious Disease in the Blood Supply and the Public Health Response." *Seminars in Hematology* 43 (2 supplement 3) (Apr 2006): S4–S9.

Farley, Thomas A. "Sexually Transmitted Diseases in the Southeastern United States: Location, Race, and Social Context." *Sexually Transmitted Diseases* 33 (7 Supplement) (July 2006): S58-64.

Fauci, A. S. "The Acquired Immune Deficiency Syndrome. The Ever-Broadening Clinical Spectrum." *Journal of the American Medical Association* 249 (1983): 2375–76.

"Finally Free to Speak Plainly?" *FrontPage*, June 26, 1992, 1, 9.

Fischer-Krentz, Jeri. "Grants Awarded to Support Black Community—First Round of Aid Goes to 3 Local Groups." *Charlotte Observer*, December 5, 1995, 2C.

Fiscus, S. A., A. A. Adimora, V. J. Schoenbach, W. Lim, R. McKinney, D. Rupar, J. Kenny, C. Woods, and C. Wilfert. "Perinatal HIV Infection and the Effect of Zidovudine Therapy on Transmission in Rural and Urban Counties." *Journal of the American Medical Association* 275 (19) (May 15, 1996): 1483–88.

Fitzsimon, Chris. "Evelyn Foust on Combating AIDS in NC." NC Policy Watch: Radio Interviews, December 8, 2008, http://www.ncpolicywatch.com/cms/2008/12/08/evelyn-foust-on-combatting-aids-in-nc. May 20, 2010.

———. "The Life-Threatening Budget Cuts." NC Policy Watch, March 16, 2010, http://www.ncpolicywatch.com/cms/2010/03/16/the-life-threatening-budget-cuts/. May 20, 2010.

"Folksinger's Tunes to Help Raise Funds for AIDS Houses." *Raleigh News & Observer*, October 3, 1991, F3.

Ford, Chandra, Kathryn Whetten, Susan Hall, Jay Kaufman, and Angela Thrasher. "Black Sexuality, Social Construction, and Research Targeting 'The Down Low' ('The DL')." *Annals of Epidemiology* 17 (3) (2007): 209–16.

Fordyce, E. J., S. Sambula, and R. Stoneburner. "Mandatory Reporting of Human Immunodeficiency Virus Testing Would Deter Blacks and Hispanics from Being Tested." *Journal of the American Medical Association* 262 (1989): 349.

Foust, Evelyn. "Call to Action: HIV/AIDS and STDS in the South." *EpiNotes* 4 (2002): 1–2, 3.

Frame, Randy. "The Church's Response to AIDS: Is Compassion Waning in Light of a So-Called Gay Disease?" *Christianity Today*, November 22, 1985, 50.

Frey, William H. "The New Great Migration: Black Americans' Return to the South, 1965–2000." *The Brookings Institution, The Living Cities Census Series*. Washington, D.C.: The Brookings Institution, May 2004.

Friedman, P., and T. Joslin. *Silverlake Life - The View from Here*. New York, Zeitgeist Films, 1993.

Fulghum, James. "AIDS: Testing and Reporting." *North Carolina Medical Journal* 51 (4) (April 1990): 143–44.

Fullilove, R. E., M. T. Fullilove, B. P. Bowser, and S. A. Gross. "Risk of Sexually Transmitted Disease among Black Adolescent Crack Users in Oakland and San Francisco, Calif." *Journal of the American Medical Association* 263 (1990): 851–55.

Funk, Tim. "Chairmen Let Many Bills Die — New Deadlines Inspire Grumbling." *Charlotte Observer*, May 29, 1987.

———. "N.C. Health Officials Hedge on AIDS Rule." *Charlotte Observer*, November 14, 1987, 1B.

Gallo, Robert C. *Virus Hunting: Aids, Cancer, and the Human Retrovirus: A Story of Scientific Discovery*. New York: Basic Books, 1994.

Garfield, Ken. "Charlotte AIDS Fight Targets Black Ministers." *Charlotte Observer*, November 20, 1995, 1C.

———. "New Year's Eve Given a Sacred Flavor." *Charlotte Observer*, December 30, 1995, 2G.

Garloch, Karen. "AIDS: Delta Wants Money Cut for AIDS Agency." *Charlotte Observer*, May 5, 1988, 7C.

———. "AIDS Agency, Others Still Wait for N.C. to Distribute U.S. Grants." *Charlotte Observer*, June 27, 1988, 1B.

———. "AIDS Fear Rivals Cancer, Heart Ills." *Charlotte Observer*, August 13, 1987, 1A.

———. "AIDS Infighting Doctor's Diplomacy Brought Down the Battle Lines in Mecklenburg." *Charlotte Observer*, March 13, 1989, 1A.

———. "AIDS Needs Aren't Being Addressed in N.C., Support Groups Complain." *Charlotte Observer*, June 8, 1990, 2C.

———. "AIDS Network Wins Grant." *Charlotte Observer*, June 20, 1994, 1E.

———. "AIDS Project Keeps Step with Disease." *Charlotte Observer*, June 15, 1987, 1A.

———. "AIDS Report Focuses on Attitude, Education." *Charlotte Observer*, March 8, 1989, 1A.

———. "AIDS Virus Casts Deadly Shadow, Abuses of Youth Plague Woman." *Charlotte Observer*, December 1, 1990, 1A.

———. "Clause on Housing Cut from AIDS Bill." *Charlotte Observer*, July 30, 1987, 3C.

———. "Congregations Reach out in an AIDS Ministry that Offers . . . a Human Touch." *Charlotte Observer*, November 10, 1994, 1C.

———. "County, AIDS Group Get $29,500 Grant." *Charlotte Observer*, August 19, 1988.

————. "Judge: Anonymous AIDS Testing Stays." *Charlotte Observer*, September 1, 1994, 1C.

————. "Kooyman Rejected for Panel: AIDS Project Director Not on Task Force." *Charlotte Observer*, February 25, 1988, 1C.

————. "N.C. AIDS Plan Apparently Unique, Officials Say." *Charlotte Observer*, October 30, 1987, 4E.

————. "N.C. Law Requires Doctors to Report AIDS-Virus Victims." *Charlotte Observer*, February 1, 1990.

————. "N.C. Legislators Debating How to Attack AIDS." *Charlotte Observer*, May 11, 1987, 1A.

————. "N.C., 9,000 Test Positive for HIV." *Charlotte Observer*, December 3, 1996, 1C.

————. "Plan for Tackling AIDS under Attack." *Charlotte Observer*, October 29, 1987, 1A.

————. "Some MDs Push More AIDS Tests." *Charlotte Observer*, April 2, 1989, 1A.

————. "United AIDS Effort Urged to Prolong, Improve Lives." *Charlotte Observer*, February 8, 1991, 1B.

Gauthier, Candace Cummins. "HIV Testing, Informed Consent, and Confidentiality." *North Carolina Medical Journal* 52 (11) (November 1991): 558–62.

Gebo, K. A., J. A. Fleishman, R. Conviser, E. D. Reilly, P. T. Korthuis, R. D. Moore, J. Hellinger, P. Keiser, H. R. Rubin, L. Crane, F. J. Hellinger, W. C. Mathews, and the HIV Research Network. "Racial and Gender Disparities in Receipt of Highly Active Antiretroviral Therapy Persist in a Multistate Sample of HIV Patients in 2001." *Journal of Acquired Immune Deficiency Syndromes* 38 (1) (2005): 96–103.

General Assembly of North Carolina. Ratified Bill. 1993 Session. Chapter 321, Senate Bill 27.

————. 1993 Session. Senate Bill 695/House Bill 738.

————. 1995 Session. Chapter 534, House Bill 834.

Gilman, Sander. *Disease and Representation: Images of Illness from Madness to AIDS*. Ithaca, N.Y.: Cornell University Press, 1988.

Gladwell, Malcolm. "New Victims, Problems Mark 10th Anniversary of AIDS." *Raleigh News & Observer*, June 5, 1991, 4A.

Glendy, Bob. "People with AIDS Share Pain, Insight with Strategy Group." *Charlotte Observer*, May 12, 1990, 6F.

Goldstein, Richard. "AIDS and Race: The Hidden Epidemic." *Village Voice*, March 10, 1987.

Golin, Carol, Frederick Isasi, Jean Breny Bontempi, and Eugenia Eng. "Secret Pills: HIV-Positive Patients' Experiences Taking Antiretroviral Therapy in North Carolina." *AIDS Education and Prevention* 14 (4) (2002): 318–29.

Gorbach, P. M., B. P. Stoner, S. O. Aral, W. L. Whittington, and K. K. Holmes. "'It Takes a Village': Understanding Concurrent Sexual Partnerships in Seattle, Washington." *Sexually Transmitted Diseases* 29 (2002): 453–62.

Gostin, Lawrence O. "Public Health Law in an Age of Terrorism: Rethinking Individual Rights and Common Goods." *Health Affairs* 21 (6) (2002): 79–93.

Governor's Crime Commission. "Crime and Justice in North Carolina: An Examination of 1984–1994 Data and Trends." North Carolina Department of Crime Control and Public Safety, n.d., http://www.gcc.state.nc.us/trends.htm. January 10, 2006.

Graves, Bill. "AIDS Curriculum adopted by State Board of Education." *Raleigh Times*, December 3, 1987.

———. "Board of Education OKs Revised AIDS Curriculum." *Raleigh Times*, December 4, 1987.

Gutis, Philip S. "Attacks on U.S. Homosexuals Held Alarmingly Widespread." *New York Times*, June 8, 1989, A24.

Guttentag, M., and P. Secord. *Too Many Women: The Sex Ratio Question*. Beverly Hills: Sage, 1983.

Hale, Grace Elizabeth. "'For Colored' and 'For White': Segregating Consumption in the South." In *Jumpin' Jim Crow: Southern Politics from the Civil War to Civil Rights*, edited by Jane Dailey, Glenda Elizabeth Gilmore, and Bryant Simons, 162–82. Princeton, N.J.: Princeton University Press, 2000.

Halperin, Edward. "Informed Consent for AIDS Testing; Or, Whose Vein Is It Anyway?" *North Carolina Medical Journal*, 51 (4) (April 1990): 145–49.

Hammonds, Evelynn M. "Missing Persons: African-American Women, AIDS and the History of Disease." *Radical America*, 24 (2) (April–June 1990): 7–24.

———. "Seeing AIDS: Race, Gender, and Representation." In *The Gender Politics of HIV/AIDS*, edited by N. Goldstein and J. L. Manlowe, 113–26. New York: New York University Press, 1997.

Harrison, Beth. "LGHP Ends Search for Director." *FrontPage*, August 11, 1995, 1, 7.

Harrison, R. J., and D. H. Weinberg. "How Important Were Changes in Racial and Ethnic Residential Segregation between 1980 and 1990?" *Proceedings of the Social Statistics Section*, 1992.

He, W., S. Neil, H. Kulkarni, E. Wright, B. K. Agan, V. C. Marconi, M. J. Dolan, R. A. Weiss, S. K. Ahuja. "Duffy Antigen Receptor for Chemokines Mediates Trans-Infection of HIV-1 from Red Blood Cells to Target Cells and Affects HIV-AIDS Susceptibility." *Cell Host & Microbe* 4 (1) (2008): 52–62.

"Health Director Backs 'Confidential' HIV Tests." *Fayetteville Observer*, June 16, 1994.

"The Health Project Helps and Needs Help." *FrontPage*, November 20, 1984, 13.

Heckman, T. G., A. M. Somlai, J. Peters, J. Walker, L. Otto-Salaj, C. A. Galdabini, J. A. Kelly. "Barriers to Care among Persons Living with HIV/AIDS in Urban and Rural Areas." *AIDS Care* 10 (3) (1998): 365–75.

Helms, Ann Doss. "AIDS Council Faces More Cases." *Charlotte Observer*, August 7, 1988, 1.

———. "Town Meeting on AIDS Brings Requests for Help, Honesty." *Gastonia Observer*, May 18, 1990, 5.

Hey, Robert P. "Education Emphasized as Way to Prevent the Spread of AIDS." *Christian Science Monitor*, June 5, 1987.

"HIV/AIDS in Rural America." National Rural Health Association, November 1997.

"HIV/AIDS Policy Fact Sheet: The HIV/AIDS Epidemic in the United States, June 2007." Menlo Park, Calif.: Kaiser Family Foundation, July 2007, 1.

"HIV Infection to Be Monitored: Health Officials Hope to Learn More about AIDS Carriers in N.C." *Greensboro News & Record*, February 4, 1990, D3.

Ho, D. D. "Time to Hit HIV, Early and Hard." *New England Journal of Medicine* 333 (7) (August 17, 1995): 450–51.

Ho, D. D., A. U. Neumann, A. S. Perelson, W. Chen, J. M. Leonard, M. Markowitz, National Conference on Human Retroviruses and Related Infections. "Rapid Turnover of Plasma Virions and CD4 lymphocytes in HIV-1 Infection." *Nature* 373 (6510) (January 12, 1995): 123–26.

Hoar, Stephen. "Request Denied to Renew Anonymous Aids Testing." *Raleigh News & Observer*, November 16, 1991, B4.Holleran, Andrew. *Ground Zero*. New York: William Morrow & Company, 1988.

Hood, John. "State House Sweep: The Real Republican Revolution." *Reason*, February 1995, http://www.reason.com/news/show/29622.html. November 25, 2008.

Hopkins, John D. "Inspired to Dance." *Associated Press*, June 8, 1977.

Hossfeld, Leslie. "Poverty in the East, 1980–2000: What Has Changed?" Wilmington, N.C.: Eastern North Carolina Poverty Committee, 2001, http://www.povertyeast.org/toolkit/research/default.html. October 24, 2006.

Iceland, John, and Daniel H. Weinberg. *Racial and Ethnic Residential Segregation in the United States: 1980–2000*. U.S. Census Bureau, Census Special Report, CENSR-4, Washington, D.C.: U.S. Government Printing Office, 2002.

The Impact of AIDS in North Carolina: A Strategic Response. Raleigh: HIV Consortia, March 19, 1993.

Irwin, D. E., J. C. Thomas, P. A. Leone et al. " Sexually Transmitted Disease Patients' Self-Treatment Practices Prior to Seeking Medical Care." Abstract K74. In *Abstracts of the 35th Interscience Conference on Antimicrobial Agents and Chemotherapy (San Francisco)*. Washington, D.C.: American Society for Microbiology, 1995.

Jaffe, H. W., K. Choi, P. A. Thomas, H. W. Haverkos, D. M. Auerbach, M. E. Guinan, M. F. Rogers, T. J. Spira, W. W. Darrow, M. A. Kramer, S. M. Friedman, J. M. Monroe, A. E. Friedman-Kien, L. J. Laubenstein, M. Marmor, B. Safai, S. K. Dritz, S. J. Crispi, S. L. Fannin, J. P. Orkwis, A. Kelter, W. R. Rushing, S. B. Thacker, and J. W. Curran. "National Case-Control Study of Kaposi's Sarcoma and Pneumocystis Carinii Pneumonia in Homosexual Men: Part 1. Epidemiologic Results." *Annals of Internal Medicine* 99 (2) (August 1983): 145–51.

Jaffe, Jody. "AIDS: As Epidemic Spreads, So Does the Fear." *Charlotte Observer*, June 8, 1983.

———. "Looking for a Common Thread among Risk Groups." *Charlotte Observer*, June 8, 1983.

Jameson, Tonya. "Delivering a Message about AIDS — Play to Deal with Disease's Effect on the Black Community." *York [S.C.] Observer*, December 1, 1995, 1Y.

"John Singleton Copley Tour: Watson and the Shark, 1778, Object 8 of 12." Wash-

ington, D.C.: National Gallery of Art, http://www.nga.gov/collection/gallery/
gg60b/gg60b-46188.0.html. June 2, 2010.

Johnston, Flo. "Black Churches to Join in AIDS Awareness Week." *Durham Herald-Sun*, March 2, 1996, B1.

Jolly, David. "About the Lesbian/Gay Health Project." *FrontPage*, May 24, 1983.

———. "AIDS: Information for North Carolina Legislators." Division of Health
Services, North Carolina Department of Human Resources, AIDS Program
(1987).

———. "Extension of Deadline for AIDS Education Projects Targeting Minority
Communities." North Carolina Department of Human Resources, February 25,
1988. Howard Fitts Personal Collection, Durham, N.C.

———. "Howard Fitts Letter, September 6, 1989." North Carolina Department of
Human Resources, 1989. Howard Fitts Personal Collection, Durham, N.C.

———. "HTLV-III: To Test or Not to Test?" *FrontPage*, May 21, 1985.

———. "Lesbian and Gay Heath Project." *Lesbian and Gay Health Project Newsletter*,
June 1984.

———. "To the Readers of The FrontPage." *FrontPage*, September 27, 1983.

Jones, Alison. "State Loses AIDS Test Suit." *Raleigh News & Observer*, June 2, 1993, B2.

Jones, James H. *Bad Blood: The Tuskegee Syphilis Experiment*. New York: Free Press,
1993.

Jones, Jim. "AIDS Effort Under Way: Support Network Opens Statewide." *Raleigh
News & Observer*, October 6, 1991, C1.

Juhasz, Alexandra. "The Contained Threat: Women in Mainstream AIDS Documentary." *Journal of Sex Research* 29 (1) (February 1990): 25–46.

Kaiser Commission on Medicaid and the Uninsured. *The Medicaid Resource Book*.
Menlo Park, Calif.: Kaiser Family Foundation, 2003.

Kaiser Family Foundation. "Sexually Transmitted Diseases in America: How Many
Cases and at What Cost?" www.kff.org/womenshealth/1445-Std Rep3.cfm.
February 7, 2006.

Kaiser Family Foundation, National Alliance of State and Territorial AIDS Directors, and the Southern State AIDS Directors Work Group. "Southern States
Summit on HIV/AIDS and STDs: A Call to Action." Keynote Address by Dr.
David Satcher, Charlotte, N.C., November 14, 2002. Menlo Park, Calif.: Kaiser
Family Foundation, 2002, 3. http://www.kaisernetwork.org/health_cast/
uploaded_files/kff111401_keynote.pdf. May 18, 2010.

Kanigel, Rachele. "Activists Seek Anonymous AIDS Testing." *Raleigh News & Observer*,
November 5, 1991, B2.

———. "Continued Anonymity in AIDS Tests Urged." *Raleigh News & Observer*,
January 16, 1991, B1.

———. "New Rule Could End AIDS Test Anonymity." *Raleigh News & Observer*,
January 13, 1991, A1.

———. "State Places Limits on Anonymous Tests: Angry AIDS Activists Lash out at
Commission." *Raleigh News & Observer*, February 13, 1991, A1.

Katz, Dolly. "Scientists Link Stress, Hypertension in Blacks." *Charlotte Observer*, April 17, 1987, 19A.

Kegeles, S. M., J. A. Catania, T. J. Coates, L. M. Pollack, and B. Lo. "Many People Who Seek Anonymous HIV-Antibody Testing Would Avoid It under Other Circumstances." *AIDS* 4 (1990): 585–87.

Kegeles, S. M., T. J. Coates, B. Lo, and J. A. Catania. "Mandatory Reporting of HIV Testing Would Deter Men from Being Tested." *Journal of the American Medical Association* 261 (1989): 1275–76.

Kelley, Colleen F., Christina M. R. Kitchen, Peter W. Hunt, Benigno Rodriguez, Frederick M. Hecht, Mari Kitahata, Heide M. Crane, James Willig, Michael Mugavero, Michael Saag, Jeffrey N. Martin, and Steven G. Deeks. "Incomplete Peripheral CD4$^+$ Cell Count Restoration in HIV-Infected Patients Receiving Long-Term Antiretroviral Treatment." *Clinical Infectious Diseases* 48 (2009): 787–94.

Keshavjee, S., S. Weiser, and A. Kleinman. "Medicine Betrayed: Hemophilia Patients and HIV in the US." *Social Science & Medicine* 53 (8) (October 2001): 1081–94.

Kilmarx, P. H., A. A. Zaidi, J. C. Thomas, A. K. Nakashima, M. E. St. Louis, M. L. Flock, and T. A. Peterman. "Ecologic Analysis of Socio-Demographic Factors and the Variation in Syphilis Rates among Counties in the United States, 1984–93." *American Journal of Public Health* 87 (1997): 1937–43.

King, J. L., and K. Hunter. *On the Down Low: A Journey into the Lives of 'Straight' Black Men Who Sleep with Men.* New York: Broadway Books, 2004.

Kirkpatrick, Christopher. "Cost of AIDS Drugs Becoming Health Emergency." *Durham Herald-Sun*, December 14, 1997, C1.

———. "Drugs Elusive for 22 Here with HIV." *Durham Herald-Sun*, December 14, 1997, A2.

Kirp, David L. *Learning by Heart: AIDS and Schoolchildren in America's Communities.* New Brunswick, N.J.: Rutgers University Press, 1989.

Kitahata, M. M., T. D. Koepsell, R. A. Deyo, C. L. Maxwell, W. T. Dodge, and E. H. Wagner. "Physicians' Experience with the Acquired Immunodeficiency Syndrome as a Factor in Patient's Survival." *New England Journal of Medicine* 334 (1996): 701–6.

Kitahata, M. M., S. E. Van Rompaey, and A. W. Shields. "Physician Experience in the Care of HIV-Infected Persons Is Associated with Earlier Adoption of New Antiretroviral Therapy." *Journal of Acquired Immune Deficiency Syndromes* 24 (2) (2000): 106–14.

Koop, C. Everett. "Surgeon General's Report on Acquired Immune Deficiency Syndrome." Washington, D.C.: U.S. Public Health Service, 1986.

Kramer, Larry. *The Normal Heart.* New York: Plume Publishing, 1990.

———. *Reports from the Holocaust: The Making of an AIDS Activist.* New York: Saint Martin's Press, 1998.

Kretzschmar, M., and M. Morris. "Measures of Concurrency in Networks and the Spread of Infectious Disease." *Mathematical Biosciences* 133 (1996): 165–95.

Kushner, Tony. *Angels in America: A Gay Fantasia on National Themes*. Parts 1 and 2. New York: Theatre Communications Group, 1993.

Lam, N., and K. Liu. "Spread of AIDS in Rural America, 1982–1990." *Journal of Acquired Immune Deficiency Syndromes* 7 (5) (1994): 485.

Lamme, Robert. "Care Lags Behind AIDS' Pace." *Fayetteville Observer*, February 8, 1997, SS.

———. "Protease Inhibitor 'Brew' Offers Hope." *Fayetteville Observer*, February 9, 1997.

Landis, S. E., V. J. Schoenbach, D. J. Weber, M. Mittal, B. Krishan, K. Lewis, and G. G. Koch. "Results of a Randomized Trial of Partner Notification in Cases of HIV Infection in North Carolina." *New England Journal of Medicine* 326 (2) (January 9, 1992): 101–6.

Laumann, Edward O., and Yoosik Youm. "Racial/Ethnic Group Differences in the Prevalence of Sexually Transmitted Diseases in the United States: A Network Explanation." *Sexually Transmitted Diseases* 26 (5) (May 1999): 250–61.

Lavalle, Janelle. "Internal Conflicts Challenge LGHP." *FrontPage*, June 6, 1989, 11.

———. "Women in the AIDS Movement Face Criticism from Within and Without." *FrontPage*, March 1989.

Legal Guide. Research Triangle Park, N.C.: North Carolina Gay Advocacy Legal Alliance, 2007, http://www.ncgala.org/guide/Legal_Guide.htm. November 23, 2007.

Lekus, Ian. "Health Care, the AIDS Crisis, and the Politics of Community: The North Carolina Lesbian and Gay Health Project, 1982–1996." In *Modern American Queer History*, edited by Allida Black, 227–52. Philadelphia, Pa.: Temple University Press, 2001.

Levenson, Jacob. *The Secret Epidemic: The Story of AIDS and Black America*. New York: Pantheon Books, 2004.

Lewin, Tamar. "Rights of Citizens and Society Raise Legal Muddle on AIDS." *New York Times*, October 14, 1987, A1.

Lichtenstein, B. "Stigma as a Barrier to Treatment of Sexually Transmitted Infection in the American Deep South: Issues of Race, Gender and Poverty." *Social Science & Medicine* 57 (12) (2003): 2435–45.

Lichtenstein, Bronwen, Edward W. Hook III, and Amit K. Sharma. "Public Tolerance, Private Pain: Stigma and Sexually Transmitted Infections in the American Deep South." *Culture, Health & Sexuality* 7 (1) (2005): 43–57.

Lovely, Sandra. "CO-99–12 Population Estimates for County by Age, Race, Sex, and Hispanic Annual Time Series, July 1, 1992." U.S. Census Bureau, http://statelibrary.dcr.state.nc.us/iss/NC_data/Durham1992.html. February 9, 2006.

Luloff, A. E., Michael K. Miller, and Lionel J. Beaulieu. "Social Conservatism: Determinants and Structural Stability Over Time." *Journal of Rural Studies* 2 (1) (1986): 9–18.

Lynn, Richard. "Race Differences in Sexual Behavior and Their Demographic Implications." *Population and Environment* 22 (1) (September 2000): 73–81.

Mackenzie, Sonja. "Scientific Silence: AIDS and African Americans in the Medical Literature." *American Journal of Public Health* 90 (7) (July 2000): 1145–46.

Mainous, A. G., and S. C. Matheny. "Rural Human Immunodeficiency Virus Health Service Provision: Indications of Rural-Urban Travel for Care." *Archives of Family Medicine* 5 (9) (1996): 469–72.

Mainous, A. G., R. A. Neill, and S. C. Matheny. "Frequency of Human Immuno-deficiency Virus Testing among Rural U.S. Residents and Why It Is Done." *Archives of Family Medicine* 4 (1) (1995): 41–45.

Mangle, Chris, and Karen Garloch. "AIDS Project Now Offers New Services." *Charlotte Observer*, July 8, 1991, 2E.

Manuel, John. "A Looming Crisis: AIDS in the Triangle." *Spectator*, March 7, 1991, 4–6.

Marston, Cicely, and Eleanor King. "Factors that Shape Young People's Sexual Behaviour: a Systematic Review." *Lancet* 368 (9547) (November 4–10, 2006): 1581–86.

Martin, Ed. "Authority on AIDS Says Battle Raging in Public Opinion." *Charlotte Observer*, February 25, 1987, 4A.

"Martin: Policy Would Bar AIDS Discrimination." *Charlotte Observer*, February 5, 1988, 5B.

Maschal, Richard. "More Women Battle AIDS." *Charlotte Observer*, November 20, 1994, 1A.

Massey, Douglas S. "American Apartheid: Segregation and the Making of the Under-class." *American Journal of Sociology* 96 (2) (September 1990): 329–57.

McClain, Kathleen. "Candlelight Vigil Pays Tribute to AIDS Victims, Patients." *Charlotte Observer*, December 2, 1991, 1C.

———. "Migrant Workers Travel a Hard Road Following the Crops." *Charlotte Observer*, October 6, 1985, 1A.

McClain, Kathleen, and Karen Garloch. "Chambers Insists County Pull AIDS Support Group's Money." *Charlotte Observer*, January 15, 1988, 2C.

McFadden, Robert. "Judge Overturns U.S. Rule Blocking 'Offensive' Educational Material on AIDS." *New York Times*, May 12, 1992, B3.

McGovern, Theresa. "Barriers to the Inclusion of Women in Research and Clinical Trials." In *The Gender Politics of HIV/AIDS in Women*, edited by Nancy Goldstein and Jennifer L. Manlowe, 43–62. New York: New York University Press, 1997.

McKenzie, Bryan. "Health Counselors Going to Church in Battle to Fight AIDS." *Fayetteville Observer*, February 3, 1989.

McKinney, M. M. "Variations in Rural AIDS Epidemiology and Service Delivery Models in the United States." *Journal of Rural Health* 18 (3) (Summer 2002): 455–66.

———, ed. *Rural HIV/AIDS: Issues in Prevention and Treatment. Proceedings of the Southeastern Conference on Rural HIV/AIDS.* Atlanta, Ga., 1997.

McLaughlin, Nancy H. "Guilford Schools Still Reviewing Sex Ed Materials." *Greensboro News & Record*, April 7, 1996, B1.

Mitchell, Monte. "More People Learn About—and Turn to—AIDS Alliance." *Charlotte Observer*, May 22, 1996.

Montagnier, Luc. *Virus: The Co-Discoverer of HIV Tracks Its Rampage and Charts the Future*. New York: W. W. Norton, 1994, 2000.

Moore, Shirley Hunter. "Alliance's Mission: To Help, to Teach." *Charlotte Observer*, October 24, 1990, 1.

Moose, Debbie. "Women and AIDS: Women Struggling to Cope with the HIV Virus Have Largely Been Ignored." *Raleigh News & Observer*, August 2, 1992, E1.

"Morbidity and Mortality Statistics." *N.C. Health Statistics Pocket Guide—1995*. Raleigh: North Carolina Center for Health Statistics, 1995, Table 5.

Morehouse, Macon. "Calls to AIDS Hotline Jump, Study Also Shows Women More Likely to Call Than Men." *Gastonia Observer*, December 24, 1991, 1.

———. "7-County Region Gets Grant to Fight AIDS, Improve Health Care." *Charlotte Observer*, January 20, 1990, 2B.

Morris, M., and M. Kretzschmar. "Concurrent Partnerships and Transmission Dynamics in Networks." *Social Networks* 17 (1995): 299–318.

Moss, Gary. "Brush with Death Brings a New Purpose to Life." *Fayetteville Observer*, August 15, 1988.

———. "Epidemic Just Beginning to Be Felt." *Fayetteville Observer*, August 16, 1988.

———. "Faith in God Gave Solace from Fear." *Fayetteville Observer*, August 18, 1988.

Mullen, Rodger. "HIV Task Force: 'There's No Magic Bullet.'" *Fayetteville Observer*, March 13, 1988.

Mullis, Lee. "Health Project Update." *Lambda*, November–December, 1983, 10.

Nagy, John A. "Anonymous Tests Win Reprieve Panel Changes Decision." *Greensboro News & Record*, November 5, 1994, A1.

Napravnik, S., J. J. Eron, R. G. Mckaig, A. D. Heine, P. Menzes, and E. B. Quinliyan. "Factors Associated with Fewer Visits for HIV Primary Care at a Tertiary Clinic." *AIDS Care* 18 (supplement 1) (2006): S45-S50.

Neergaard, Lauran. "Officials Debate Whether HIV Patients Should Be Named in Effort to Track Cases." *Charlotte Observer*, January 28, 1993.

Neumann, M. S., and E. D. Sogolow. "Replicating Effective Programs: HIV.ASIDS Prevention Technology Transfer." *AIDS Education and Prevention* 12 (supplement A) (2000): 35–48.

"New AIDS Treatment Approved." *Raleigh News & Observer*, June 28, 1994, D8.

Nielsen, F., and A. S. Alderson. "Income Inequality, Development, and Dualism: Results from an Unbalanced Cross-National Panel." *American Sociological Review* 60 (1995): 674–701.

Nietzsche, Friedrich. *Beyond Good and Evil: Prelude to a Philosophy of the Future*. New York: Vintage, 1989.

"1990 Census of Population and Housing, North Carolina—Summary Tape File 1: Profile 1—Characteristics of the Population." U.S. Census Bureau, 1990.

1990 Census of Population and Housing, Summary Tape File 3: Poverty Status. Raleigh: North Carolina Office of State Planning, September 14, 1992, 19.

North Carolina AIDS Advisory Council. *The NC/AIDS Index.* Raleigh: AIDS Care
Branch, North Carolina Department of Environment, Health, and Natural
Resources, 1996.

North Carolina AIDS Program. *AIDS: Information for North Carolina Legislators.*
Raleigh: North Carolina Department of Human Resources, February 1987.

North Carolina Department of Health and Human Services, Division of Public
Health, Communicable Disease Branch. *N.C. Epidemiologic Profile for HIV/STD
Prevention and Care Planning.* Raleigh: North Carolina Department of Heath
and Human Services, 2009.

North Carolina Department of Health and Human Services, Division of Public
Health, HIV/STD Prevention and Care Branch. *N.C. Epidemiologic Profile for
HIV/STD Prevention and Care Planning.* Raleigh: North Carolina Department of
Health and Human Services, 2005.

———. "Chapter 5: Special Studies." In *N.C. Epidemiologic Profile for HIV/STD
Prevention and Care Planning*, 65–66. Raleigh: North Carolina Health and
Human Services, 2005.

———. "Get Real. Get Tested." Raleigh: North Carolina Department of Health
and Human Services, November 17, 2009, http://www.epi.state.nc.us/epi/hiv/
grgt.html. May 20, 2010.

———. *N.C. Epidemiologic Profile for HIV/STD Prevention and Care Planning*, Raleigh:
North Carolina Health and Human Resources, 2007.

North Carolina Department of Health and Human Services. "North Carolina HIV
Cases." N.d.

———. "State-Wide Community Conference on AIDS, Greensboro, NC, August
28–29, 1987." Raleigh: North Carolina Department of Human Resources,
August 1987.

"North Carolina Doctors to Report AIDS." *FrontPage*, September 6, 1983.

Nussbaum, Bruce. *Good Intentions: How Big Business and the Medical Establishment
Are Corrupting the Fight against AIDS, Alzheimer's, Cancer, and More.* New York:
Penguin Books, 1990.

Oleske, James, Anthony Minnefor, Roger Cooper Jr., Kathleen Thomas, Antonio dela
Cruz, Houman Ahdieh, Isabel Guerrero, Vijay V. Joshi, and Franklin Desposito.
"Immune Deficiency Syndrome in Children." *Journal of the American Medical
Association* 249 (1983): 2345–49.

Oppenheimer, Gerald. "In the Eye of the Storm: The Epidemiological Construction
of AIDS." In *AIDS: The Burdens of History*, edited by Elizabeth Fee and Daniel
M. Fox, 267–300. Berkeley: University of California Press, 1988.

Ortiz-Torres, Blanca, Irma Serrano-García, and Nélida Torres-Burgos. "Subverting
Culture: Promoting HIV/AIDS Prevention among Puerto Rican and Dominican Women." *American Journal of Community Psychology* 28 (2000): 859–81.

Paddock, Polly. "Project Would Give AIDS Victims Last Home." *Charlotte Observer*,
January 15, 1990, 1D.

———. "Save Lives: Keep AIDS Test Secret." *Charlotte Observer*, January 28, 1991, 1B.

Palella, Frank J., Jr., Maria Deloria-Knoll, Joan S. Chmiel, Anne C. Moorman,

Kathleen C. Wood, Alan E. Greenberg, Scott D. Holmberg, and the HIV Outpatient Study (HOPS) Investigators. "Survival Benefits of Initiating Antiretroviral Therapy in HIV-Infected Persons in Different CD4$^+$ Cell Strata." *Annals of Internal Medicine* 138 (2003): 620–26.

Patton, Cindy. *Inventing AIDS*. New York: Routledge, 1990.

Pear, Robert. "U.S. Files First AIDS Discrimination Charge." *New York Times*, August 9, 1986.

Perrow, Charles, and Mauro F. Guillen. *The AIDS Disaster: The Failure of Organizations in New York and the Nation*. New Haven, Conn.: Yale University Press, 1990.

Peterson, J. L., and G. Marin. "Issues in the Prevention of AIDS among Black and Hispanic Men." *American Psychologist* 43 (11) (November 1988): 871–77.

Piot, Peter. "AIDS: The Impact of Other Sexually Transmitted Diseases." *Network* 9 (2) (Winter 1988): 4.

Popovic, M., M. G. Sarngadha, Elizabeth Read, and Robert Gallo. "Detection, Isolation, and Continuous Production of Cytopathic Retroviruses (HTLV-III) from Patients with AIDS and Pre-AIDS." *Science* 224 (4648) (May 4, 1984): 497–500.

Porterfield, Deborah, Genevieve Dutton, and Ziya Gizlice. "Cervical Cancer in North Carolina: Incidence, Mortality, and Risk Factors." *North Carolina Medical Journal* 64 (1) (January/February 2003): 11–17.

Poulsen, P. A. "Alkyl Nitrite as an Aphrodisiac." *Ugeskr Laeger*, July 18, 1983, 145.

Poverty and Health Statistics Branch/HHES Division. *Current Population Survey, Annual Social and Economic Supplements*. Washington, D.C.: U.S. Bureau of the Census, 2007, http://www.census.gov/hhes/www/poverty/histpov/hstpov1.html. May 28, 2010.

"Pregnancy and Outcome Statistics." *N.C. Health Statistics Pocket Guide — 1995*. Raleigh: North Carolina Center for Health Statistics, 1995, Table 4.

Pressley, Sue Anne. " . . . Another's Frightening Future: Stricken Durham Man and His Lover Learn to Live in Death's Shadow." *Charlotte Observer*, June 5, 1983, 1, 11.

————. "One Victim's Final, Horrible Days." *Charlotte Observer*, June 5, 1983.

Pride, Don, and Ted Mellnik. "N.C. Bill Would Deny Licenses for Marriage to AIDS Carriers." *Charlotte Observer*, February 19, 1987, 1A.

"Prisons Fear Start of AIDS Epidemic." *Greensboro News & Record*, July 23, 1990, B2.

Pullen, Lisa. "Autrey Reverses Stance, Backs AIDS Group." *Charlotte Observer*, February 12, 1988, 1D.

Quigley, Kathryn. "AIDS Finds Victims with Rural Address." *Fayetteville Observer*, August 19, 1995.

Rapp, James. "Innovative Projects Focusing on the Prevention of AIDS." Paper presented at the An Awareness of Cultural Norms and Values: The Black Community's Response to AIDS. Health Sciences Building, North Carolina Central University, Durham, N.C., October 10, 1988.

Ready, Tinker. "Judge Halts Plan to End Anonymous AIDS Tests." *Raleigh News & Observer*, September 1, 1994, A1.

———. "New Drugs Brighten Prognosis for AIDS: Experts Optimistic but Still Cautious." *Raleigh News & Observer*, February 2, 1997, A1.

Reale, Robin L. "HIV Class Plays to Students' Interests." *Chapel Hill Herald*, December 16, 1996, 3.

Recer, Paul. "Study: Drugs Other Than AZT May Be More Effective in AIDS Fight." *Charlotte Observer*, September 15, 1995, 5A.

Reif, Susan, Kathryn Whetten, and Nathan Theilman. "Association of Race and Gender with Use of Antiretroviral Therapy among HIV-Infected Individuals in the Southeastern United States." *Southern Medical Journal* 100 (8) (August 2007): 775–81.

Rene, Norman. *Longtime Companion*. USA: MGM, 1990.

Rengert, G. F. *The Geography of Illegal Drugs*. Boulder, Colo.: Westview Press, 1996.

"Request for Application (RFA) for Funds for Community-Based HIV/STD Risk Reduction Prevention Projects, January 20, 1993." *HIV/STD Control Branch*. Raleigh: North Carolina Department of Environment, Health, and Natural Resources, 1993, 2.

Resnicow, K., R. Braithwaite, J. Ahluwalia, and T. Baranowski. "Cultural Sensitivity in Public Health: Defined and Demystified." *Ethnicity and Disease* 9 (1) (1999): 10–21.

Rhee, Foon. "Hunt's Agenda." *Charlotte Observer*, February 14, 1993, 6C.

Rhee, Jong Mo. "The Redistribution of the Black Work Force in the South by Industry." *Phylon* 35 (3) (1974): 293–300.

Richissin, Todd. "This Corner Is the End of the Road." *Raleigh News & Observer*, December 6, 1993, A1.

Ricketts, T. *Rural Health in the United States*. New York: Oxford University Press, 1999.

"Roberts Honored by Dominican Republic President." *University Gazette*, October 9, 2002, http://gazette.unc.edu/archives/02oct09/facstaff.html. December 3, 2007.

Robertson, Tricia. "AIDS Is Equal-Opportunity Killer, Program Tells Blacks." *Wilmington Morning Star*, April 15, 1987, 2C.

Robinson, Isaac. "Blacks Move Back to the South." *American Demographics* 8 (1986): 40–43.

Rogers, Martha, and Walter W. Williams. "AIDS a Big Problem among Blacks, Hispanics." *Wilmington Morning Star*, April 3, 1987.

"The Role of the Church in AIDS Education and Prevention." *DCI Clearinghouse and Network Center*, June 29, 1989, Howard Fitts Personal Collection, Durham, N.C.

Rose, Dina R., and Todd R. Clear. "Incarceration, Social Capital and Crime: Implications for Social Disorganization Theory." *Criminology* 36 (1998): 441–79.

Rosenbrock, Rolf, Francoise Dubois-Arber, Martin Moers, Patrice Pinell, Doris Schaeffer, and Michel Setbon. "The Normalization of AIDS in Western European Countries." *Social Science & Medicine* 50 (11) (June 2000): 1607–29.

Ross, Jill. "Anonymous Testing of AIDS Will Continue." *Charlotte Observer*, January 5, 1993, 2C.

Rounds, K. A. "AIDS in Rural Areas: Challenges to Providing Care." *Social Work* 33 (1988): 257–61.

Rowe, M. J., and C. C. Ryan. "Comparing State-Only Expenditures for AIDS." *American Journal of Public Health* 78 (4) (April 1988): 424–29.

Rumley, Richard L. "The Future of a Futureless Future." *PICalif.SO Newsletter* 2 (3) (July/August 1994): 1.

Rumley, R. L., N. C. Shappley, L. E. Waivers, and J. D. Esinhart. "AIDS in Rural Eastern North Carolina–Patient Migration: A Rural AIDS Burden." *AIDS* 5 (11) (1991): 1373–78.

Rushton, J. P. *Race, Evolution, and Behavior.* New Brunswick, N.J.: Transaction, 1995.

Russell, Christine. "Immunity Systems Linked to Ailment Afflicting Gay Men." *Washington Post*, December 11, 1981, A2.

"SCDAP to Implement Program for HIV-AIDS." *Greensboro News & Record*, July 31, 1996, 7.

Schable, B., T. Diaz, and J. W. Ward. "The Epidemiology of HIV in the Rural South." Paper presented at the Eleventh International Conference on AIDS, Vancouver, Canada, 1996.

Schewel, Steve. "Carl Wittman, 1943–1986." *Independent*, January 31, 1986.

Schmalz, Jeffrey. "Whatever Happened to AIDS?" *New York Times Magazine*, November 28, 1993.

Schoenwald, Jonathan M. *A Time for Choosing: The Rise of Modern American Conservatism.* New York: Oxford University Press, 2001.

"Schools Must Teach Abstinence." *FrontPage*, August 11, 1995, 1, 7.

Schultz, Mark. "AIDS House Brimming with Health: Treatment's Success Bodes Change in Mission." *Chapel Hill Herald*, May 18, 1997, 3.

Seymore, Kelly B. "AIDS Testing Change Barred, Judge Overrules Anonymity Limit." *Raleigh News & Observer*, January 5, 1993, A1.

Shapiro, M. F., S. C. Morton, D. F. McCaffrey, J. W. Senterfitt, J. A. Fleishman, J. F. Perlman, L. A. Athey, J. W. Keesey, D. P. Goldman, S. H. Berry, and S. A. Bozzette. "Variations in the Care of HIV-Infected Adults in the United States." *Journal of the American Medical Association* 281 (1999): 2305–15.

Shepard, Charles E. "Experts Weigh AIDS Risk to Blood Recipients." *Charlotte Observer*, June 8, 1983.

Shilts, Randy. *And the Band Played On: Politics, People, and the AIDS Epidemic.* New York: Penguin Books, 1988.

"Sickle Cell Grant." *Greensboro News & Record*, November 24, 1996, 21.

Simon, Bryant. "Race Reactions: African American Organizing, Liberalism, and White Working-Class Politics in Postwar Sought Carolina." In *Jumpin' Jim Crow: Southern Politics from the Civil War to Civil Rights*, edited by Jane Dailey, Glenda Elizabeth Gilmore, and Bryant Simons, 239–59. Princeton, N.J.: Princeton University Press, 2000.

Simpson, Dave. "Wake to Offer Tests to Protect Blood Supply from AIDS." *Raleigh Times*, May 13, 1985.

Smith, Christian. *Christian America? What Evangelicals Really Want*. Berkeley: University of California Press, 2002.

Smith, David Barton. *Health Care Divided: Race and Healing a Nation*. Ann Arbor: University of Michigan, 1999.

Smith, L. S., D. Gentry. "Migrant Farm Workers' Perceptions of Support Persons in a Descriptive Community Survey." *Public Health Nursing* 4 (1) (March 1987): 21–28.

Snow, A. C. "Opinion of the Times: Tell AIDS Contacts, Too." *Raleigh Times*, September 23, 1985.

Soderberg, Kema. "Black Churches Urged to Join Fight on AIDS." *Raleigh News & Observer*, October 4, 1987, 33A, 42A.

Southern AIDS Coalition. *Southern States Manifesto: Update 2008, HIV/AIDS and Sexually Transmitted Diseases in the South*. Birmingham, Ala.: Southern AIDS Coalition, July 21, 2008.

———. *2009–2010 HIV/AIDS Health Care Policy Brief and Recommendations*. Birmingham, Ala.: Southern AIDS Coalition, 2009.

Southern State AIDS Directors Work Group. *Southern States Manifesto: HIV/AIDS and STDs in the South, A Call to Action!* Atlanta, Ga.: Centers for Disease Control and Prevention, 2003.

Southern State AIDS/STD Directors Work Group. "Southern States Manifesto: HIV/AIDS and STDS in the South: A Call to Action." National Alliance of State and Territorial AIDS Directors, March 2, 2003, 16.

Spivey, Angela. "2." *Endeavors* 24 (1) (Winter 2004), http://old-endeavors.unc.edu/win2004/hiv.html. May 28, 2009.

Spohn, Lawrence. "Officials Want AIDS Test to Be Separate from Blood Drives." *Greensboro News & Record*, March 5, 1985, B1.

State v. Richardson. 308 N.C. 470, 302 S.E.2d 799 (1983).

Steadman, Tom. "N.C. Leads Neighbors in New HIV Cases." *Greensboro News & Record*, December 3, 1996, A1.

Steffen, Monika. "The Normalisation of AIDS Policies in Europe: Patterns, Path Dependency and Innovation." In *AIDS in Europe: New Challenges for the Social Sciences*, edited by Jean-Paul Moatti et al., 207–22. New York: Routledge, 2000.

Stengel, Richard, Mary Cronin, and Steven Holmes. "The Changing Face of AIDS." *Time Magazine*, August 17, 1987, 12–14.

Stephens, Cinde. "Adopting AIDS Child Proves Hard." *Greensboro News & Record*, September 9, 1990, A1.

———. "United Way Shows AIDS Group Isn't Just for Gays." *Greensboro News & Record*, September 29, 1991, D1.

Stillwaggon, Eileen. *AIDS and the Ecology of Poverty*. New York: Oxford University Press, 2006.

Stocking, Ben. "Black Pastors Being Recruited for Fight against AIDS." *Raleigh News & Observer*, March 5, 1996, B1.

Stowe, Gene. "AIDS Test Anonymity in Question: Union County Board Recommends Change." *Charlotte Observer*, February 4, 1989, 1B.

Sugrue, Thomas J. *The Origins of the Urban Crisis: Race and Inequality in Postwar Detroit*. Princeton, N.J.: Princeton University Press, 1998.

Sullivan, Gerard. "A Bibliographic Guide to Government Hearings and Reports, Legislative Action, and Speeches Made in the House and Senate of the United States Congress on the Subject of Homosexuality." *Journal of Homosexuality* 10 (1–2) (Fall 1984): 163.

"Suspected AIDS Victim Spent Time in 10 Other Jails." *Raleigh Times*, June 1, 1983.

Taylor, Jody. "Legislator Criticizes Failure of AIDS Bills." *Charlotte Observer*, May 31, 1987, 2B.

Teachout, Leo J. "Consider HIV Testing in Terms of Public Health." *Greensboro News & Record*, January 13, 1991, E3.

Tescher, Jennifer. "Syphilis Cases Today, AIDS Cases Later? County Seeks Expertise Before Syphilis Outbreak Turns into Wave of AIDS Disease." *Charlotte Observer*, January 27, 1993, 1.

Tesoriero J. M., H. B. Battles, K. Heavner, S. Y. Leung, C. Nemeth, W. Pulver, and G. S. Birkhead. "The Effect of Name-Based Reporting and Partner Notification on HIV Testing in New York State." *American Journal of Public Health* 98 (4) (April 2008): 728–35.

Thomas, J. C. "From Slavery to Incarceration: Social Forces Affecting the Epidemiology of Sexually Transmitted Diseases in the Rural South." *Sexually Transmitted Diseases* 33 (7 Supplement) (2006): S6–10.

Thomas, J. C., and M. E. Gaffield. "Social Structure, Race, and Gonorrhea Rates in the Southeastern United States." *Ethnicity & Disease* 13 (2003): 362–68.

Thomas, J. C., A. Kulik, V. S. Schoenbach, and D. Weiner. "Syphilis in the South: Rural Rates Surpass Urban Rates in North Carolina." *American Journal of Public Health* 85 (1995): 1119–22.

Thomas, J. C., V. J. Schoenbach, G. Eng, and M. A. McDonald. "Rural Gonorrhea in the Southeastern United States: A Neglected Epidemic?" *American Journal of Epidemiology* 143 (1996): 269–77.

Thomas, J. C., and K. K. Thomas. "Things Ain't What They Ought to Be: Social Forces Underlying Racial Disparities in Rates of Sexually Transmitted Diseases in a Rural North Carolina County." *Social Science & Medicine* 49 (8) (October 1999): 1075–84.

Thomas, J. C., and E. Torrone. "Incarceration as Forced Migration: Effects on Selected Community Health Outcomes." *American Journal of Public Health* 96 (10) (October 2006): 1762–65.

Thomas, S. B., and S. C. Quinn. "The Tuskegee Syphilis Study, 1932 to 1972: Implications for HIV Education and AIDS Risk Education Programs in the Black Community." *American Journal of Public Health* 81 (1991): 1498–1505.

Toler, Laura J. "AIDS Battle Here May Call For More Funds, Education." *Raleigh Times*, November 1, 1986, 1, 9.

Tonry, Michael H. *Malign Neglect: Race, Crime, and Punishment in America*. New York: Oxford University Press, 1992.

Trew, Lucinda. "AIDS: The Gay Community Faces a Time of Crisis." *Fayetteville Observer*, June 23, 1985.

Tucker, M. B., and R. J. Taylor. "Demographic Correlates of Relationship Status among Black Americans." *Journal of Marriage and Family* 51 (1989): 655–65.

Turner, B. J., and J. K. Ball. "Variations in Inpatient Mortality for AIDS in a National Sample of Hospitals." *Journal of Acquired Immune Deficiency Syndromes* 5 (10) (1992): 978–87.

United Press International. "Falwell Urging Action to Halt Spread of AIDS." *Raleigh Times*, July 13, 1983.

U.S. Department of Justice, Office of Justice Programs, Office of Juvenile Justice and Delinquency Prevention. "Evaluation of the Disproportionate Minority Confinement (DMC) Initiative North Carolina Final Report." Prepared by Caliber Associates, May 8, 1996.

"US Finds Discrimination in Firing of AIDS Victim." *Wall Street Journal*, August 11, 1986.

Valdiserri, Ronald O., ed. *Dawning Answers: How the HIV/AIDS Epidemic Has Helped to Strengthen Public Health*. New York: Oxford University Press, 2003.

———. "HIV/AIDS' Contribution to Community Mobilization and Health Planning Efforts." In *Dawning Answers: How the HIV/AIDS Epidemic Has Helped to Strengthen Public Health*, edited by Ronald O. Valdiserri, 56–75. New York: Oxford University Press, 2003.

———. "HIV/AIDS in Historical Profile." In *Dawning Answers: How the HIV/AIDS Epidemic Has Helped to Strengthen Public Health*, edited by Ronald O. Valdiserri, 3–32. New York: Oxford University Press, 2003.

Vanderbush, Patience. Personal communication with author, Durham, N.C., October 4, 2006.

Vauaghan, John. "Hello, AIDS Hotline? I'm Afraid . . ." *Charlotte Observer*, January 4, 1987, 1E.

Verghese, Abraham. *My Own Country: A Doctor's Story*. New York: Vintage Books, 1994.

Wallace, Rodrick. "A Synergism of Plagues: 'Planned Shrinkage,' Contagious Housing Destruction, and AIDS in the Bronx." *Environmental Research* 47 (1) (October 1988): 1–33.

Warden, Billy. "Activists Bemoan Scarcity of Blacks in AIDS Effort." *Raleigh News & Observer*, April 21, 1992, A1.

Wasserheit, J. N. "Epidemiological Synergy. Interrelationships between Human Immunodeficiency Virus Infection and Other Sexually Transmitted Diseases." *Sexually Transmitted Diseases* 19 (2) (March–April 1992): 61–77.

Weatherford, Carole Bosto, and Ronald J. Weatherford, *Somebody's Knocking at Your Door*. Binghamton, N.Y.: Haworth Pastoral Press, 1998.

Weber, D. J., W. A. Rutala, G. P. Samsa, F. A. Sarubbi Jr., and L. C. King. "Epidemiology of Tuberculosis in North Carolina, 1966 to 1986: Analysis of Demographic Features, Geographic Variation, AIDS, Migrant Workers, and Site of Infection." *Southern Medical Journal* 82 (10) (October 1989): 1204–14.

Weinberg, P. D., J. Hounshell, L. A. Sherman, J. Godwin, S. Ali, C. Tomori, and C. L. Bennett. "Legal, Financial, and Public Health Consequences of HIV Contamination of Blood and Blood Products in the 1980s and 1990s." *Annals of Internal Medicine* 136 (4) (February 19, 2002): 312–19.

Weslowski V. B., D. P. Andrulis, and V. Martin. *AIDS in Rural America*. Baltimore, Md.: National Public Health and Hospital Institute, 1992.

Whetten-Goldstein, Kathryn, and Trang Quyen Nguyen. *"You're the First One I've Told": New Faces of HIV in the South*. New Brunswick, N.J.: Rutgers University Press, 2003.

Whetten-Goldstein, Kathryn, T. Q. Nguyen, and A. E. Heald. "Characteristics of Individuals Infected with the Human Immunodeficiency Virus and Provider Interaction in the Predominantly Rural Southeast." *Southern Medical Journal* 94 (2) (2001): 212–22.

White, Katherine. "Most Children with AIDS Seen as No Threat in Classroom." *Charlotte Observer*, January 21, 1986.

White, Ryan, and Ann Marie Cunningham. *Ryan White: My Own Story*. New York: Signet, 1991.

White, Sharon E. "Living in the Shadow of AIDS: Faith and Support Buoy Victims, Their Loved Ones." *Charlotte Observer*, March 10, 1996, 1L.

———. "A Week of Prayer for AIDS Healing." *Charlotte Observer*, March 8, 1996, 1L.

Whiteley, Michael. "Two More Inmates May Be AIDS Victims." *Raleigh Times*, May 30, 1983.

Whyte, B. M., and J. C. Carr. "Comparison of AIDS in Women in Rural and Urban Georgia." *Southern Medical Journal* 85 (6) (1992): 571–78.

Wilkie, Lorry. "Minorities Offered AIDS Education." *Fayetteville Observer*, July 14, 1992.

Williams, Rhonda Y. "AIDS Test Proposal Attacked, Dropping Anonymity Dangerous, Critics Say." *Charlotte Observer*, January 24, 1991, 1D.

Wilson, Bonnie. "AIDS in County Rise by 57%." *Fayetteville Observer*, January 8, 1994.

———. "Dogwood Consortium." *Fayetteville Observer*, February 14, 1994.

Wilson, Chip. "Gaston Seeks Battle Plan against AIDS." *Charlotte Observer*, February 24, 1988, 1.

Wilson, W. J. *The Truly Disadvantaged: The Inner City, the Underclass, and Public Policy*. Chicago: University of Chicago Press, 1987.

———. *When Work Disappears: The World of the New Urban Poor*. New York: Random House, 1996.

Wise, Janet. "Focus Group of Gay/Bisexual Male HIV Prevention Educators." Raleigh: HIV/STD Control Branch, February 8, 1993.

Wittman, Carl. *Refugees from Amerika: A Gay Manifesto*. San Francisco: Free Press, 1970.

Wohl, D. A., L. Shain, M. Adamian, B. L. Stephenson, R. Strauss, C. Golin, and A.

Kaplan. "HIV Transmission Risk Behaviors among HIV-Infected Individuals Released from Prison." Conference on Retroviruses and Opportunistic Infections, February 10–14, 2003, Abstract no. 36.

Womble, Jeffery. "AIDS Awareness." *Fayetteville Observer*, October 14, 1995.

———. "Program Provides Fun and Education." *Fayetteville Observer*, February 15, 1992.

———. "Taking It to the Streets: AIDS Educator Dispenses Compassion and Condoms." *Fayetteville Observer*, September 12, 1991.

Youngblood, Karen. "AIDS Story Is Survival, Victim Says." *Fayetteville Observer*, July 28, 1989.

Zaleski, E. H., and K. M. Schiaffino. "Religiosity and Sexual Risk-Taking Behavior during the Transition to College." *Journal of Adolescence* 23 (2000): 223–27.

Zepp, Carol. "Durham HIV Clinic to Expand Services." *Durham Herald-Sun*, November 3, 1991, B1.

Zimmer, Jeff. "Activists Angry over HIV Testing Decision." *Durham Herald-Sun*, February 11, 1995, A8.

———. "Activists, N.C. Officials Meet in Court to Battle over Anonymous HIV Tests." *Durham Herald-Sun*, May 18, 1995, C1.

———. "AIDS Funding Evades State Budget Cuts." *Durham Herald-Sun*, July 5, 1995, C1.

———. "AIDS Moving Up on List of County's Top Killers, Now 4th." *Durham Herald-Sun*, January 19, 1997, A2.

———. "Anonymous HIV Testing Gets Reprieve: N.C. High Court Eyes Appeal." *Durham Herald-Sun*, August 1, 1996, C1.

———. "Anonymous HIV Testing Heading to State Supreme Court." *Durham Herald-Sun*, January 21, 1997, C1.

———. "Board: Condoms Worth the Cost." *Durham Herald-Sun*, February 10, 1995, C8.

———. "Court Ends Anonymous Test for HIV." *Durham Herald-Sun*, July 17, 1996, C1.

———. "Court Ruling Spells End to Anonymous HIV Testing: Durham Activist Group Says Decision Denies Public's Right to Privacy." *Durham Herald-Sun*, April 12, 1997, A1.

———. "Housing Situation Often Tenuous for Durham's AIDS/HIV Sufferers: Money Often Goes for Treatment Rather than Place to Live." *Durham Herald-Sun*, January 24, 1996, C8.

———. "N.C. Supreme Court to Rule on HIV Testing: Health Officials Want to End Anonymity." *Durham Herald-Sun*, September 12, 1996, C1.

———. "Science Brings Hope to Day Marking Fight against AIDS: Drug Cocktail Stops Virus, but Education Still Target." *Durham Herald-Sun*, December 1, 1996, B1.

Zimmerman, Jonathan. *Whose America? Culture Wars in the Public Schools.* Cambridge, Mass.: Harvard University Press, 2002.

INDEX

North Carolina Memorial Hospital, 28, 30, 40, 45
Noto, Dante, 31–32
Nucleic acid amplification tests (NAAT), 1

Opportunities Industrialization Center, 59
Orange County, 93

Page, Colin, 76
Partner notification, 77, 87–88
Patronage sex, 96
Piedmont AIDS Consortium, 115
Pierson, Terry, 111
Pitt County, 99, 103
Pneumocystis carinii pneumonia, 14, 26, 111
Politicization of AIDS, 47
Poverty, HIV/AIDS and, 15, 23, 40, 44, 63, 80, 99, 100, 103–4, 106, 109, 135; in rural communities, 103, 106
Presidential campaign, 2008, 123
Prisons, HIV/AIDS and, 67, 87, 91
Privette, Coy, 47–49, 134
Project First Step, 59
Project Straighttalk, 54–55, 131
Protease inhibitors, 110, 124

Quarantine: AIDS added to quarantine law, 151 (n. 23); gays' fear of, 35; suggested as AIDS prevention method, 48, 105
Quigless, Milton D., 79

Raleigh, HIV/AIDS in, 1, 53, 55, 59, 78, 80
Regional AIDS Consortium, 61
Regional AIDS Interfaith Network (RAIN), 60
Rein, Barbara, 86
Republican administration, HIV policy and, 76, 78, 99, 115
Republicans, 47, 75–76, 89
Risk factors, individual, 9, 62, 79, 91, 101, 125
Robeson County, 60
Rocky Mount, 59, 73
Rowand, Glenn, 13–14, 21, 27–28
Rozier, Ashley, 112
Rumley, Richard, 97, 99–100, 102–6, 109–10, 112, 127, 132, 135–36

Rural communities, HIV/AIDS and, 5, 45, 51, 67, 95, 97, 99, 102–3, 106–7, 113, 118, 125, 136, 163 (n. 60), 164 (n. 80); health care infrastructure and, 45, 112; minorities and, 97, 99, 102–3;
Rutherford, Carlton, 68
Ryan White Comprehensive AIDS Resources Emergency (CARE) Act, 61, 92–93, 103, 109, 114, 120–22, 133
Ryan White HIV/AIDS Treatment Modernization ACT (RWHATMA), 121–22; and Eligible Metropolitan Areas, 122

Sachs, Susan, 115
Screening and Tracing of Active Transmission (STAT) Team, 1
Sex, safer, 50, 90, 96, 125; transactional, 64–65, 96, 132
Sex education, 47, 50, 89–90; abstinence and, 47, 89, 115, 150 (n. 19)
Sex ratios, 22, 67 Sexual concurrency, 16, 24, 27, 65–66, 68, 100–101, 132, 146 (n. 6), 155 (n. 48); separational, 24, 66
Sexually transmitted infection (STI), HIV and, 15–16, 22, 28, 121, 142 (n. 19), 144 (n. 61)
Sexual minorities, 100, 131
Sexual networks, 16, 22–23, 63, 65–66; racialized segregation of, 22, 65–66, 69, 144 (n. 62)
Sexual violence, HIV/AIDS and, 101
Sex workers, 48
Shanti Project, 29, 32
Shaw University, 53
Sickle Cell Disease Association, 117
Smiley, Lynn, 33–34, 45–46
Smith, Mark, 80
Social conservatives, 11, 47, 50, 73, 90–92, 115–16, 132–34
Social determinants of health, 23, 62–63, 66, 80, 91–92, 99, 132, 135, 137
Social Security Disability Insurance (SSDI), 31–32, 60
Southern AIDS Coalition, 121–23; support of opt-out testing by, 123
Southern Baptists, 60